Be

Mainstream

Medicine

Beyond Mainstream Medicine

Dialogue towards a new paradigm for health

Thomas Hardtmuth
Richard House

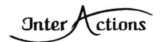

Published at the same time in German as
*Verständigung: Ein medizinisch - psychologischer Dialog
über natürliche Immunität*
Amthor Verlag, 2022
with changes for the English edition

English edition published by
InterActions
Stroud, UK

©InterActions 2022
www.interactions360.org
contact@interactions360.org

ISBN 978-0-9528364-8-3

Layout and front cover design by InterActions;
rear cover design - see Acknowledgements

Printed in the UK
by ImprintDigital.com

Contents

Preface

With their publication, *Beyond Mainstream Medicine*, Thomas Hardtmuth and Richard House have presented a small masterpiece for which one can only be grateful. For here, not only does a committed doctor and deep expert in virology come to an understanding with a humanistic psychologist and developmental researcher about the Corona pandemic experience and what one could learn from it so far. But one also understands why the complexity of the pandemic and the type of media coverage could polarise society so profoundly, even in family contexts, and what thoughts and perspectives are now needed to heal the psychosocial and economic after-effects and collateral damage that have arisen.

No therapy without a clear diagnosis!

And both are conveyed by the introductory chapters and the subsequent engaging and true-to-life dialogue between the two experts. Theoretical medical, virological, financial and economic factors are explained in a generally understandable way, as is the connection with the omnipresent ecological crisis and the serious downsides of our current increasingly commercial and profit-oriented health care system. Particularly inspiring is the clear description of a necessary paradigm shift in medicine, in which each and every one of us can actively participate. For at the centre of this new paradigm for health is the individual human being with his or her special possibilities to strengthen his or her spiritual, soul and physical health and thus his or her complex immune system. Such knowledge calms fears, deepens trust in destiny and gives courage to constructively meet the challenges of our present time.

Michaela Glöckler
June 2022

Foreword

This extended dialogue between psychologist Richard House and medical physician Thomas Hardtmuth originally began as an open interview for an English magazine, but in the course of time it developed into an animated, mutual exchange that far exceeded the initially planned scope. As a result, the text was first published as a book in German in the Spring of 2022, under the title *Verständigung: Ein medizinisch-psychologischer Dialog über natürliche Immunität* (a fairly literal translation of which is *Understanding through Conversation: A Medical–Psychological Dialogue on Natural Immunity*. The German edition was translated by Thomas Hardtmuth, and included an extensive introduction. In this subsequent English-language edition, the text is largely identical to the German edition, apart from some minor additions and changes made to the extended introduction.

This collaboration between Thomas and Richard arose in the context of their respective published writings on the subject of Corona. In order to provide an orientation in relation to these writings and the authors' interests and commitments, the dialogue is preceded by a contextualising introduction.

The topics treated here are based on two academic lifetimes of reading and research, and therefore on numerous literature sources, the more important of which are listed in the extensive notes and bibliography sections. A complete, 'academic' listing of all our sources would go beyond the scope of what is intended to be an informed yet non-academic discursive conversation. Any questions with regard to references and literature sources can of course be directed to the authors via the publisher.

Thomas Hardtmuth & Richard House

July 2022

Introduction:
Corona in Context

Thomas Hardtmuth, with Richard House

The Corona crisis is far more than just a virus problem. Rather, it is an enormous challenge for the development of global consciousness. Uncertainty, controversy and fear, even anger and aggression, are arising worldwide at the present time. But completely new questions are also emerging: there is intensive discussion, argument and writing, with completely new communication structures and networks forming that more and more seem to be replacing the established media.

It is part of the nature of a crisis – and a characteristic of 'liminality' – that the old is not yet overcome and the new is not yet clearly in sight – a generally valid principle of individual as well as social development. There are phases during which difficulties, challenges and a certain level of disorientation occur, drawing forth a commitment to master the issues, and ultimately often emerging from the crisis strengthened and with newly forged insights and abilities.

In his *Faust*, Goethe lets the creator speak: 'Man's activity can all too easily slacken, He soon loves himself the unconditional rest; Therefore I gladly give him the journeyman, Who irritates and works and must create as a devil.' (Faust I, *Prologue in Heaven*) In Goethe's sense, then, evil in the world is not only there to deceive and seduce people, but it is *a wake-up call* given to us by the Creator Himself. We could not make a free decision for the good if evil did not exist. Without the devil we would sleep through the good: we would not even notice it, just as without the experience of darkness we would not develop an awareness of the light. And without death, we would not even ask the question about the meaning of life.

We can make it clear with an example from *Genesis*. In the Garden of Eden, the serpent appears as the embodiment of evil, and tempts Eve to eat from the tree of knowledge. With the serpent, the poison appears that we need as human beings in order to be able to discern and recognise in an independent way. Just as humans ingest all kinds of poisons to make themselves artificially more alert (caffeine, nicotine, alcohol and various drugs), they also physiologically have poison-related substances in their brains so that they can think independently. The messenger substances in our brain, the so-called neurotransmitters, are related to poisons. The venom of the hornet, for example, contains almost all the neurotransmitters of our central nervous system: Dopamine, adrenaline, histamine, serotonin, acetylcholine, etc. Without these substances, we would have no waking consciousness. That which harms us on the one hand, by learning to master and acquire it, is transformed into a new ability – 'a part of that power which always wills evil and always creates good'.

In this context, the Corona crisis can be seen as an event that, on the one hand, brings much confusion, chaos and countless conflicts, but on the other hand can be understood as a wake-up call that shakes up our consciousness and sharpens our view for necessary cognitive processes in present times.

The Corona crisis can be understood as a summation effect of developments that are problematic in intellectual history and society, the consequences of which are currently building up like several waves into a kind of tsunami.

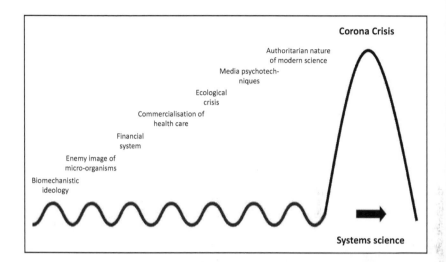

The current challenge is a fundamental shift in consciousness brought about by globalisation and the necessary learning processes associated with it. It is not only the growing awareness of our Earth as a living whole that is increasingly emerging in the face of the environmental crisis and other global socio-ecological problems, for this new way of thinking also demands an integral view of the sciences, without which perspective we will no longer be able to manage in the future. Today we speak of 'systems science', by which we mean a multi-perspectival view of all the interrelated fields. This new science overcomes the old division into natural science and the humanities. It not only works analytically by breaking things down and thinking it can discover the cause of the whole in the individual, but it seeks an understanding of complex systemic interactions, as the latter are characteristic of all living processes. This ranges from the

13

highly differentiated and diverse exchange processes of micro-organisms among themselves to modern human communication structures with all their risks and opportunities. Systems science, then, is a holistically oriented, trans-disciplinary science.

In the anthroposophical context we speak of the Age of the Consciousness Soul in which we are currently living, understanding this to mean the awakening of the soul to itself. So we begin to question ourselves: how do I actually think, how do I come to my judgements, have I really understood the thing I am advocating or am I just repeating what I have been told? In science, for example, this means epistemological self-reflection and also a historical awareness of how the various views have developed – and above all, the honest admission of all the things that we just don't know. In a time when 'knowing better' and being 'right' are becoming ever louder and more strident, there is something socially salutary about the joint realisation of our many unanswered questions.

By way of introduction, we would like to briefly outline the aspects referred to in the above diagram in order to provide an orientation framework for the topics that we discuss in the long dialogue that forms the centrepiece of this book.

Biomechanistic Ideology

The living system is exactly the opposite of a machine, in which the structure of the product depends critically on the rigidly pre-programmed operations of the individual parts. In a living system, the structure of the whole determines the action of the parts.

Paul Alfred Weiss[1]

1. Paul Alfred Weiss (1898–1989), Austrian-American biologist. He contributed significantly to systems theory and introduced a field theory to embryology.

14

The epistemological foundations of today's natural science, and thus also of virology, go back to the French philosopher René Descartes (1595–1650), who divided the human mind (*res cogitans*) and the human body (*res extensae*) in a dualistic worldview. In his time, the microscope, calculating machine, clock, printing press, spinning wheel, etc. were invented – i.e. people learned for the first time to translate mechanistic principles into technical innovations. Enormous fascination emanated from and accompanied these new possibilities. Just as digitalisation and Artificial Intelligence (AI) research are today tempting some fanatical contemporaries to stoop to transhumanist visions of life in a purely virtual world, Descartes, in the heat of the emerging fascination with apparatuses, declared all living organisms to be machines that would function according to linear and, thus, controllable causal principles. This way of thinking was in the spirit of the age of emerging technology, which is why his philosophy was quickly accepted and spread widely.

Today, fundamentally we know very well that such naïve mechanistic ideas have long since ceased to be sufficient for understanding life and health, but nevertheless this Cartesian dualistic paradigm still dominates scientific and medical habits of thought – not least because the entire medical and pharmacological industrial complex owes its profitable existence to the dogma of technological controllability. Only the idea of a kind of uniform 'body machinery' is capable of legitimising standardised therapy concepts such as vaccinations, which are uniformly administered to billions of people worldwide under the idea of uniformly functioning immune systems. But it is precisely the example of our highly individual immune system that makes it clear how crucial a holistic, i.e. systems-science approach, is for understanding immune functions.

'We don't yet understand too much about how the whole immune defence system works', says Professor Mark Morris Davis, molecular biologist and immunologist from Stanford University, California.

The functional connections and interrelatedness of our immune functions with the brain and nervous system, with our gut microbiome, our lifestyle and our entire psychosocial environment, are so complex and multi-layered that the common, one-dimensional antigen–antibody logic is basically an inadmissible, even a criminal reductionism. Just one example will suffice here. If actors play emotionally negative scenes with violence, fear and hatred, a weakening of their immune functions can be directly measured in the blood; and the opposite happens in the case of humorous scenes.[2] Humour, trust, fairness, co-operation, concentration, meditation, interest, etc. have an immediate stimulating effect on the immune system, while fear, powerlessness and helplessness have a weakening effect.

The central problem of immunological research lies precisely in the *highly individual* reaction and functioning of the immune system; a mechanistic logic is incapable of explaining much here. Only an understanding of individual life circumstances and biographical experiences can adequately describe the immune functions: they are directly related to our life situation, our emotional states and long-term experiences (stress, relationships, conflicts, fears, etc.) – a phenomenon which has been convincingly demonstrated by psychoneuroimmunological research in recent years, based on numerous studies. The mere confrontation with a virus says little if anything about the cause and course of an illness, because we are constantly confronted

2.   See P. Klapps, Humor und Gesundheit – Ansichten eines Clowns [Humour and Health – Views of a Clown], mimeo; available at https://tinyurl.com/5n7jdme7 (accessed 26 June 2022).

with a multitude of potential pathogens; with every breath, we take in thousands of viruses and bacteria, without any symptoms of illness occurring.

There are three factors on which the development of an infectious disease essentially depends:

- **Constitution** (biography, individual personality traits, lifestyle, hereditary factors)
- **Disposition** (age, sex, risk factors, climate, occupation, stress, etc.)
- **Exposure** (contact with viruses and bacteria)

The decisive factor is the state of our immune system, which in turn depends upon our constitution and disposition. Chronic negative stress in particular has the most lasting effect on the immune system. In stress research, we distinguish not only psychological stressors but also physical stressors such as noise, heat, cold, radiation, etc. There is now ample data showing, for example, a close correlation between particulate matter in the air and the risk of respiratory infections such as Covid-19.[3] Similarly, several studies show a consistent link between electro-smog and various diseases: our entire organism is interspersed with bioelectrical signals, the external stimulation of which is known to have therapeutic uses, but which can also be irritated by excessive densities of ambient electromagnetic radiation, e.g. from 5G technology, and can lead to significant health disorders.[4]

Covid-19 pandemic management has almost exclusively been

3   C. Arvay, *Wir können es besser* [We Can Do Better], Quadriga-Verlag, Köln, 2020, pp 90–101.

4   D. Meijer, H. Geesink & J. Timmer, 'The 5G safety dilemma: plea for urgent scientific research in the European context', ResearchGate, mimeo, April 2020; available at https://tinyurl.com/mrxx7mma (accessed 26 June 2022).

focused on exposure, i.e. merely confronting the virus, which it wants to reduce through hygiene rules, lockdowns, masks, contact bans, etc. and has certainly not shied away from drastic interventions in civil liberties and personal rights. However, convincing results from these measures could not be achieved, as the comparison with countries (or US states) without such measures has clearly demonstrated.[5] On the contrary, the negative influences on our immune system generated by isolation, fear, loneliness, exclusion, unemployment, conflicts, relationship crises and domestic violence, and much more, are not even predictable from within their cosmology. A general weakening of human immune systems cannot be recorded at all with our usual methods of statistical data collection, because the effects of immuno-suppression through psychosocial and other forms of stress are just as complex and individual as are the people themselves. A causal connection between the symptoms of illness caused by such immuno-suppression and the aforementioned Corona measures can therefore always be denied from a narrow positivistic viewpoint, but is *de facto* present.

According to stress researcher Prof. Dr Mazda Adli of Charité Berlin, social isolation is one of the most powerful, disease-independent negative health predictors that we know of; several meta-analyses have shown that social isolation has a greater effect on premature mortality than obesity, smoking or alcohol abuse. If, for example, people currently suffer from acute episodes of autoimmune diseases (rheumatism, multiple sclerosis, inflammatory bowel diseases, childhood diabetes and many more), which are now also referred to as 'stress-associated diseases', then this is rarely associated with rising stress levels

5.   Regarding the effectiveness of lockdowns, see J. Herby, L. Jonung & S.H. Hanke, 'A literature review and meta-analysis of the effects of lockdowns on Covid-19 mortality', *Studies in Applied Economics*, 200, January 2022; available at https://tinyurl.com/uv7bmp2t (accessed 26 June 2022).

stemming from all the intervening Corona measures.

The old biomechanistic understanding of disease, then, largely misses the reality of people's lives due to its one-dimensional view, no longer corresponding to the state of knowledge of modern integrative medicine.

I think that the analogy between cells and machines is misleading and misplaced. Such a mechanistic approach has not been able to help us understand the complexity of life processes and will not do so in the future.

Thomas C. G. Bosch[6]

The Enemy Image of Micro-organisms

Viruses are the never-ending front of evolution.... They continually shape the trajectory of life on the planet, including that of humans.

Luis Villarreal[7]

Insights into the human microbiome and its multi-layered relationships with our organism have only become clearer in recent years. The approximately 40 trillion microbes that live in symbiosis with us are essential for numerous healthy functions, including our psychological well-being. The microbiome is now understood as an organ of the human being. Viruses are also important components of this organ; there are about ten viruses for every bacterium, but their role in the system of microbial processes is still largely misunderstood. We only know that viruses, as the primordial building blocks of life, play an important

6.   See Bosch, 2017, p. 20. Thomas Bosch is Professor of General Zoology at the University CAU Kiel.
7.   Luis Villarreal, 'A life in viruses', 13 May 2016, Rita Allen Foundation; available at https://tinyurl.com/47k5m8dc (accessed 26 June 2022). Luis Villarreal is Professor at the University of California, Irvine, at the Center for Virus Research, Department of Molecular Biology and Biochemistry.

role in the regulation of population dynamics – that is, in the correct composition of the individual microbiome. The 'fight against the viruses' (note the telling military metaphor) can thus also become a fight against *one's own organism*, and may possibly play a certain role in the development of immunologically caused pathologies such as autoimmune diseases (referred to below).

When Robert Koch isolated the first micro-organisms from the bodily secretions of sick people in the nineteenth century, a new image of the enemy was born, and he declared *'war against the smallest but most dangerous enemies of the human race'*.[8] At that time, researchers had no idea about the vital functions or 'organ nature' of the microbiome. A real 'military campaign' began – the Charité was a military hospital – with countless antibacterial strategies and products. However, these procedures, some of which were indeed undoubtedly helpful, also had their downsides. Since the mass use of antibiotics, disinfectants, vaccinations, fever suppositories, etc., a whole new disease profile has developed, especially in the industrialised nations. Modern diseases such as allergies, autoimmune diseases and cancer, which have been steadily on the rise for about 70 years, are ultimately based on irritations of the immune systems that are related to an increasing loss of microbiome diversity. In the case of cancer, the immune system reacts too weakly, in the case of allergies too strongly, and in the case of autoimmune diseases (of which there are now some 80 different ones), it attacks its own organism. In the Western industrial nations, some 30 per cent of people suffer from allergies; in the USA there are 50 million autoimmune patients (equivalent to 15 per cent of the population); and in Germany one in four people dies of cancer.

8.   Lecture at the Charité University Hospital in Berlin on 4 August 1890 about bacteriological research, in front of numerous physicians from all over the world.

Amongst the peoples of less 'developed' countries, all these diseases are much rarer.

The connection between declining infectious diseases, on the one hand, and a simultaneous increase in immunologically caused diseases, has been known since the 1980s, but this has generally not yet been realised. The key role of the microbiome in these modern diseases is not yet widely understood. A huge industry still thrives on, and has a strong vested interest in, the 'war' against viruses and bacteria. Antibiotics are among the most widely prescribed substances of all. They can be justified in certain cases, but are often prescribed out of fear or ignorance, not because they make medical sense. The oft-heard claim that the decline in infectious diseases is a success of vaccinations and antibiotics does not correspond to the facts. Overall infectious disease mortality had already fallen by some 90 per cent *before* the first antibiotics came on to the market and mass vaccinations were introduced.

The decline in death rates for scarlet fever, diphtheria, whooping cough, and measles in children under 15 years of age show that from 1860 - 1955 mortality decreased by 90% before the introduction of vaccination and antibiotics.
Ivan Illich (Illich, 1976)

The continuous decline in infectious mortality since the middle of the nineteenth century was primarily due to the improvement of living conditions (housing, warm clothing, sufficient food, clean drinking water, heating, light, hygiene, social security and much more), and the reduction of stress (cold, poverty, confinement, hunger, existential fear, etc.). As living conditions improved, so did people's natural immune functions. Epidemics have essentially largely disappeared in countries with humane living and hygiene standards, but the old fears relating to viruses and bacteria have remained.

The fear of new killer viruses (SARS, MERS, bird flu, swine flu), which has been stoked again and again in recent years, is experiencing a high point in the current Corona crisis, but the actual mortality data speak against the justification of such fears, and above all against the exaggerated forecasts that are regularly spread at the beginning of such waves of infection. In the UK, the wildly inaccurate forecasts of disgraced epidemiologist Professor Neil Ferguson have become a cultural figure of fun and the butt of many a joke. In Germany, we even had a *lower* mortality rate in the Corona year 2020,[9] which is not really expected during a pandemic. If higher mortality rates are reported from other countries, this must very likely have other reasons and cannot be due to the virus, because it is the same everywhere and, as we know, the virus knows no national borders. For an epidemiological analysis, it is very difficult to differentiate between the causes of death caused by the virus and those caused by the multiple measures taken against it (including inappropriate, iatrogenic treatment protocols). In general, the commonly heard assertion that a person 'died of a virus' basically amounts to inadmissible reductionism, because the death of a person is always a multi-layered event and is connected with numerous other factors.

Financial System

Hunger kills about 100,000 people a day worldwide. Hardly anyone talks about this genocide, let alone remedies. Against this background and in the face of the rampant neoliberalism of the financial markets, the talk of the powerful

9. B. Kowall, F. Standl, F. Oesterling & others, 'Excess mortality due to Covid-19? A comparison of total mortality in 2020 with total mortality in 2016 to 2019 in Germany, Sweden and Spain', *Plos One*, 3 August 2021; available at https://tinyurl.com/bdfy3n7j (accessed 26 June 2022).

about Christian values, solidarity and justice is exposed as
pure hypocrisy.

Jean Ziegler[10]

Errors can only be maintained for a while, but at some point they have to be corrected, otherwise they grow to monstrous dimensions.

In 1990, the trading volume of the entire global real economy was 22 trillion dollars and that of the financial economy about 2 trillion, so trading on the capital market accounted for about one tenth of the real economy. In 2016, this ratio had already reversed, with the real economy's trading volume amounting to 73 trillion dollars, and trading in derivatives ten times that amount, at 705 trillion dollars.[11] The real producing economy has thus become a mere appendage of the financial economy.

As long as the banking system fulfils its actual profession, for example to transparently invest money deposits of savers in meaningful projects, it also has a meaningful task for society as a whole. If, however, money itself becomes a commodity that is only traded according to strategies of profit maximisation, ignoring people's needs, money becomes an end in itself and, from a systems theory point of view, what we call a carcinoma in the organism, a proliferation, develops. Financial flows no longer go where they are beneficial to the social organism

---

10. Jean Zieger is a sociologist who has taught at the universities of Geneva and Paris. He was a member of the Swiss Parliament from 1981 to 1999. Until 2008, he was UN Special Rapporteur on the Right to Food. He is known for his statement that 'A child who dies from hunger is a murdered child'.

11. See Deutscher Bundestag, Wissenschaftliche Dienste [German Bundestag, Scientific Services], 'Dokumentation: Zu den Begriffen Finanz- und Realwirtschaft' [Documentation: On the terms financial and real economy], WD 5 – 3000 / 003/20, 2020; available at https://tinyurl.com/ycxnc2d8 (accessed 26 June 2022).

and the common good, but develop a kind of autonomous, self-propagating internal circulation in profit-oriented 'bubbles'. If the money is not invested appropriately in social and cultural projects, but mainly in the economy itself according to its tenets of profit maximisation, the result is a monstrously inflated financial world with hopeless overproduction, and the money is lacking for nurses, teachers, educators, social pedagogues, cultural workers and much more. This is indeed the current situation in which we find ourselves.

The deregulation of the financial markets in the 1970s and 1980s, mainly promoted by the governments of Margaret Thatcher in Great Britain, Ronald Reagan in the USA and Helmut Kohl in Germany, initiated a development that many economists describe as the beginning of a global madness. A concrete example may illustrate this.[12] After the bursting of the financial bubble in 2008, stock-exchange traders discovered raw materials and foodstuffs on the world market as an object of speculation, which led to the world market prices for rice, maize and grain rising within a short time, in some cases by several hundred per cent. This in turn had the consequence that millions of people were driven to the abyss of starvation. At the time, the presenter of the *Heute Journal*, Claus Kleber, was filming a documentary on the causes of global hunger,[13] and he found out that in India, football pitch-sized heaps of grain bags were rotting, serving as a speculative commodity and, in a sense, being held back from the market in order to keep prices high. At the same time, just a few hundred metres away, people lived in hunger and misery in the slums. In India, about 1 million children starve to death

12. For further discussion, see also Thomas Hardtmuth, *Medizin im Würgegriff des Profits* [Medicine in the Stranglehold of Profits], Amthor Verlag, Heidenheim, 2017.
13. See ZDFzoom: Hunger! [in German], 5 November 2014; available at https://tinyurl.com/284vyu59 (accessed 26 June 2022).

every year due to malnutrition – just one-sixth of these rotten speculative goods would have been enough to prevent this.

With the deregulation of the financial markets, a global system was created that can be reduced to the simple formula: Having money is more lucrative than working. If the returns and interest from the financial economy exceed real economic growth, i.e. if more 'cream' is skimmed off than production delivers, this cannot go well in the long run and must inevitably lead to the collapse of the system, as in the financial crisis of 2008, when the so-called 'bank bailout' swallowed up hundreds of billions of taxpayers' money that was actually intended for more sensible purposes.

According to an Oxfam study in 2022,[14] the approximately 2700 billionaires of this world have increased their wealth from 8.6 to 13.8 trillion dollars between March 2020 and November 2021; and the ten richest people have even doubled it, to 256 billion. In the same period, the number of people living in extreme poverty has increased by 163 million. The Corona measures have therefore not only divided society, but also massively promoted the widening chasm between rich and poor, and thus social injustice worldwide.

With the grotesquely growing wealth of an ever-smaller and ever more powerful financial elite, global debt has also increased almost exponentially. According to the Debt Report

---

14. See the OXFAM International report, *Inequality Kills: The Unparalleled Action Needed to Combat Unprecedented Inequality in the Wake of COVID-19*, Oxford, 17 January 2022; available at https://tinyurl.com/2p93uxa9 (accessed 26 June 2022). See also '10 Reichste Männer verdoppeln ihr Vermögen – über 160 Millionen Menschen zusätzlich in Armut' [Corona pandemic and inequality: 10 richest men double their wealth – over 160 million more people in poverty], OXFAM Publication, 17 January 2022; available at https://tinyurl.com/4r7fxxs3 (accessed 26 June 2022).

2021,[15] it currently stands at almost 300 trillion dollars – one has to ask: to whom do we owe these debts? After all, the debts of some are always the assets of others. As a result of the 'pandemic management', the debt crisis has worsened massively, especially in the Southern Hemisphere, which inevitably increases the dependence of countries on the power elites of the financial world and thus their ability to be blackmailed.

With many of the supposedly unexpected happenings that are unfolding in world politics today, we should always ask ourselves who is earning from it. The Corona crisis has generated trillions in profits; the Ukraine crisis is now the beginning of a new stage in the global armament madness; and Western energy companies, especially the US fracking gas and oil industry, are rubbing their hands because the cheap Russian energy supplies to Europe have now largely been stopped, thus providing an argument for driving up prices without restraint. It is only from the perspective of economic strategies that some current events take on a certain logic.

If this social carcinoma of finance and profit mania is not treated, further global crises will inevitably follow. The central problem can be characterised thus: if the organs of cultural and intellectual life become venal – i.e. if, for example, fewer and fewer people own ever-growing media empires in addition to their business enterprises – then there is a growing danger that influencing public opinion will become part of business strategies and will thus destroy a central element of any healthy community of life – viz. its diversity. Moreover, this applies to biological ecosystems just as much as it does to social communities. Where diversity is lost, pathological monocultures spread; and these are ultimately the parasitic diseases – biolog-

---

15. See *Schuldenreport 2021* [Debt Report 2021], Misereor / erlassjahr.de; available at https://tinyurl.com/mrnr85ad (accessed 26 June 2022).

ical and social. The uniformity of media opinion management during the Corona crisis provided ample opportunity to study such pathologies. We will return to this point at length in this book.

Commercialisation of Health Care

The moment care serves profit, it has lost true care.
Bernhard Lown, Nobel Peace Prize 1985

The globally deregulated financial market has created a system of speculators, investors and hedge fund managers whose investment strategies are less and less oriented towards the promotion of culture and the common good, and ever more towards pure profit maximisation. They make no contribution to society, they produce nothing and provide no services, yet they shift millions on the stock exchange within milliseconds with the help of computer algorithms – a kind of shell game trick for quick money. This system has unleashed a highly pathological frenzy of capital, the fatal consequences of which for the environment and social justice all over the planet are now becoming increasingly apparent.[16]

The fundamental systemic error committed by policy-makers in the long run-up to the Corona crisis was to declare health care a market. The fact that money is made from illness is the beginning of the end of all medical ethics. A doctor's therapeutic decisions must be radically decoupled from his or her income, just as a judge's earnings have nothing to do with the judgements he makes. At a congress in Berlin in September 2017, the former constitutional judge Siegfried Bross spoke of

---

16. See also C. Kreiß, *Profitwahn – Warum sich eine menschengerechtere Wirtschaft lohnt* [Profit mania – Why a more humane economy is worthwhile]. Tectum Verlag, Marburg, 2013.

it being incompatible with German Basic Law ('Grundgesetz') if institutions of public welfare – which in addition to hospitals also include kindergartens, schools, waterworks, public transport, etc. – are exposed to the risks of market competition.[17] A hospital is no more a commercial enterprise than a kindergarten or a police station, which do not have to make a profit.

With the increasing commercialisation of medicine, health care institutions have become one of the safest and most lucrative objects of investment. There will always be patients, and the fear of illness, pain and death is an excellent way to do business. Investigative journalists like John Pilger in the UK have shown in great detail how, almost unnoticed, the founding principles of the UK's National Health Service have been under unremitting assault from 'marketisation' and privatisation-by-stealth for many years. For years in Germany, to give a further example, the number of hospitals run by municipalities has been declining and those run by private companies have become the majority. Such hospitals not only have to care for patients, but also serve the interests of their shareholders. Of the money paid in by citizens for hospital care in Germany, between 20 and 30 per cent now ends up in the pockets of investors, and this money is correspondingly missing from real care structures. The result is a kind of regime change that has become increasingly prevalent in medical thinking in recent decades. The trend is increasingly moving away from 'talking medicine', away from care, welfare, counselling, patient proximity, the multiple 'in-

17. See Dr Siegfried Broß, 'Positionen zur Verteilungsdebatte: Das Krankenhaus – ein kommerzieller Wirtschaftsbetrieb?' Vortrag von Dr. Siegfried Broß beim 17. Bundeskongress des Bundesverbandes Deutscher Pathologen am 23. September 2017 in Berlin [Positions on the distribution debate: The hospital – a commercial Enterprise? Lecture by Dr. Siegfried Broß at the 17th Federal Congress of the Federal Association German pathologist on 23 September 2017 in Berlin], Press Agency Health, Berlin; available at https://tinyurl.com/4dvj3ebh (accessed 26 June 2022).

tangibles' of outstanding medical care, etc. towards commodi-fication and economic 'efficiency'.

The predominance of economic logic and the associated con-straints have led to the phenomenon known as 'the medical-isation of society', with more and more diagnoses, fears and lucrative therapy strategies. Social-structural problems such as burn-out and the increasing number of mental illnesses are re-defined as pharmacologically correctable disorders. The high-est rewards are given to those who are treated with high levels of technical expenditure or toxic pharmaceuticals. The cost of a single, often questionable palliative chemotherapy treatment now exceeds the average annual salary of a hospital doctor. The therapeutic and caring professions, i.e. those which see the hu-man being as the actual 'cure', are increasingly devalued in the modern health industry to a mere cost factor, and thus a risk for the balance sheets. Accordingly, despite constant bubble-like promises of improvement by politicians, we have had growing shortages in the caring professions for years.

An example may illustrate the grotesque extent to which the power of economic logic has gained hegemony in the health sector. On 22 September 2021, the German Federal Statistical Office announced that in the Corona year 2020, 2.5 million fewer patients were treated as inpatients in Germany than in the year before, which corresponds to a drop of 13 per cent.[18] At the same time, the impending collapse of the health system was propagated in a continuous media loop, with images of overcrowded intensive care units and exhausted staff dominat-ing the evening news. At the same time, however, thousands of

18. See '13 % weniger stationäre Krankenhausbehandlungen im Jahr 2020' [13 % fewer inpatient hospital treatments in 2020], Destatis – Statis-tisches Bundesamt, Pressemitteilung No. 445, 22 September 2021; availa-ble at https://tinyurl.com/24j5hz3y (accessed 26 June 2022).

intensive care beds were cut across Germany. So we had over-crowding alarmism and at the same time a significant decrease in inpatient treatments and, in parallel, a drastic reduction in beds. Is there anyone who understands this logic?

The whole picture is made even more questionable by the fact that in the same year, 2020, hospital revenues in Germany rose by 15 per cent nationwide.[19] In TH's local hospital here in Germany, 84 emergency beds were provided for Corona patients in a neighbouring congress centre, of which none was ever occupied, but the hospital received over €500 per bed and per day. This is the real perversion; instead of providing adequate care to people according to need, numerous patients in need of treatment were sent home and more money than usual was made with empty Corona beds just to keep the pandemic panic going. Very similar stories can be told from health-care services across the Western world.

There is no doubt that there are, and always have been, annual, worldwide waves of infection of varying severity. But when health becomes more and more a 'business model' (see Maio, 2014), such waves can be instrumentalised extremely profitably, as can easily be observed at present, and the increasingly unrestrained use of fear propaganda becomes the driving force of this business.

Ecological Crisis

It is the big ones who create the very big problems, not the small ones.

Leopold Kohr[20]

19. See P. Fess, R. Hanselle & C. Stolze, 'Die Pandemie der Wissenslück-en' [The pandemic of knowledge gaps], *Cicero*, No. 1, January 2022, p. 29.
20. Leopold Kohr (1909-1994) was a national economist, lawyer, political scientist, philosopher and pioneer of the environmental movement. His guiding principle was the decentralisation of social and economic organisations to a human, manageable scale. In 1983 he received the Alternative Nobel Prize

Epidemics are not an evil freak of nature. They always have their reason in abruptly occurring distortions and imbalances within natural and socio-cultural ecosystems that have developed over long periods of time. Like human cultures, biological ecosystems are highly complex, finely balanced mixed cultures with highly individual signatures.

The most reliable indicators of the global ecological crisis are global warming and the rapidly advancing extinction of species. According to current studies,[21] only 3 per cent of the land areas on our planet still have intact ecosystems with natural animal and plant diversity. According to current IMF data, more than two-thirds of the world's wildlife has been destroyed in the last 50 years,[22] and an estimated 150 species are irretrievably lost every day. The main culprits are the agro-industrial complex with its huge, pesticide-laden monocultures, over-fishing of the oceans, rainforest deforestation, factory farming and numerous other anthropogenic influences.

A study published in 2017[23] found a significant link between rainforest deforestation and the Ebola epidemics in West and Central Africa between 1976 and 2014, with the disease usually appearing within a year where clearing had previously occurred. Habitat destruction causes fruit bats to invade human

21. See Andrew J. Plumptre, Daniele Baisero, R. Travis Belote & others, 'Where might we find ecologically intact communities?' *Frontiers in Forests and Global Change*, 15 April 2021; available at https://tinyurl.com/2p88wdwc (accessed 26 June 2022).
22. See Anon, 'Mehr als zwei Drittel der Tierwelt in den vergangenen 50 Jahren vernichtet' [More than two-thirds of wildlife destroyed in the past 50 years], *Der Tagesspiegel*, 10 September 2020; available at https://tinyurl.com/meyrfxhx (accessed 26 June 2022).
23. Jesús Olivero, Julia E. Fa, Raimundo Real & others, 'Recent loss of closed forests is associated with Ebola virus disease outbreaks', *Scientific Reports*, 7, article no. 14291, 2017; available at https://tinyurl.com/yz5d7b92 (accessed 26 June 2022).

settlements and spread their viruses there. A study in the Amazon rainforest of Brazil showed that deforestation of only 4.3 per cent of the area in a given region was associated with a 48 per cent increase in the incidence of malaria.[24] The fallow clearing areas create countless puddles in the rainy area, in which the vectors of the malaria plasmodia, the Anopheles mosquitoes, multiplied rapidly. A particularly marked increase in infectious diseases such as dengue fever, Zika and yellow fever can be seen where large palm oil and other monoculture plantations have been established on the deforested rainforest areas. A 2019 meta-analysis of 34 studies in Southeast Asia found that agro-industrialised land, for example, has a four-fold increased risk of typhus infection.[25]

The prevention of future large-scale infection events (pandemics) lies largely in organic agriculture that returns to small-scale decentralised structures. As the US evolutionary biologist Robert Wallace from the University of Minnesota proved in his book *Big Farms Make Big Flu: The New Pathogens* (Campylobacter, Nipah virus, Q fever, hepatitis E and various new influenza variants), all originate from large-scale industrial agriculture.

A fundamentally important insight for a future health ecology now lies in the fact that the macro-ecological problems of our planet are reflected in the micro-ecology of the human microbiome. More than 20,000 microbiome studies in the last 20 years

24. S.H. Olson, R. Gangnon, G. Abbad Silveira & others, 'Deforestation and malaria in Mâncio Lima County, Brazil', *Emerging Infectious Diseases,* 16 (7), July 2010, pp.1108–15; available at https://tinyurl.com/54fwyvhc (accessed 26 June 2022).
25. See Torsten Harmsen, 'Forscher: Abholzung von Wäldern fördert Infektionskrankheiten' [Researchers: Deforestation promotes infectious diseases], *Berliner Zeitung*, 25 March 2021; available at https://tinyurl.com/3s555j8t (accessed 26 June 2022).

have unmistakably shown that almost all modern diseases such as cancer, metabolic disorders (diabetes, obesity, arteriosclerosis), allergies, autoimmune diseases, mental and neurodegenerative diseases (Alzheimer's, Parkinson's) are consistently linked to the loss of microbial biodiversity in our gut microbiome. In a way, our gut flora reflects the health of the external natural world.[26]

The basic rule applies to both systems: an ecosystem is healthier and more robust, the higher its biodiversity. Parasites can spread much more easily in a 10-hectare maize field than in a natural meadow that is home to hundreds of animal and plant species in every square metre. A gut microbiome with high diversity has a much broader metabolic repertoire, i.e. a wider range of responses to changing conditions. As with an ecosystem in the wild that has grown over long periods of time – a landscape with its own character – the highly individual microbiome of humans is the best protective factor against parasitic colonisation, but also against other diseases.

In a recently published study (Wilmanski et al., 2021), microbiome analysis of more than 9,000 people between the ages of 18 and 101 showed that the healthiest men and women and those with the highest life expectancy were those whose intestinal flora was highly diverse and had changed or *individualised* the most over the years.

Against this background, there are significant implications for the Corona situation. The loss of microbiome diversity, which

---

26. A detailed description of the problem can be found in Thomas Hardtmuth, *Mikrobiom und Mensch. Die Bedeutung der Mikroorganismen und Viren in Medizin, Evolution und Ökologie – Wege zu einer systemischen Perspektive* [Mikrobiom and the Human Being. The Importance of Microorganisms and Viruses in Medicine, Evolution and Ecology – Ways to a Systemic Perspective]. Salumed-Verlag, Berlin, 2021.

has been progressing for years, is being dramatically accelerated by current measures, as the Kiel microbiome researcher Thomas Bosch has shown:

> Our evolutionary history is closely linked to the constant presence of microbes. Apparently, developmental biological processes such as the differentiation of certain immune cells are therefore set up for the constant presence of signals provided by the microbiome. If these signals are missing, the corresponding developmental steps run incompletely or even incorrectly, an immune system then emerges that is incompletely composed, incorrectly regulated and potentially pathogenic. Our microbial co-inhabitants are therefore a very important factor in the development of a functional and efficient immune system... Due to hygiene measures, antibiotics and our lifestyle, microbial diversity has been decreasing more and more rapidly in recent decades. Hygiene measures in the Covid 19 pandemic are massively reinforcing this decades-long process. (Bosch, 2020)

The sensitive phase of microbiome development takes place from birth to about 3 years of age, after which the child's individual gut flora is reasonably stable. If the microbiome is imprinted incorrectly in this early phase – we refer to this as 'pathological imprinting' – this results in lifelong immune deficits, with corresponding disease dispositions. Even before considering the dire psychological and developmental impact of masked children being robbed of experiencing the essential and foundational humanity of the human face, for young children growing up in the Corona situation, masks, contact bans, hygiene rules, etc. can be expected to lead to an increase in numerous microbiome-associated diseases, because their immune systems are being put to sleep, as it were. Since 2021, we have been experiencing the first consequences, in the form of a rapid increase in child infections with the RS virus (respiratory syncytial virus),[27] a far more dangerous disease for children than that caused by coronaviruses.

Media Psycho-techniques

But beware of false prophets, which come to you in sheep's clothing, but inwardly they are ravening wolves.

(Matthew 7:15)

Through global digital networking, every smartphone owner today is integrated into a worldwide information network, which on the one hand allows almost unlimited access to what are now many billions of internet pages, videos and countless communication forums etc.; while on the other hand, we are also constantly accessible, our geographical position and our user behaviour leave traces on the internet, which are fed into algorithms and used for personalised advertising strategies and targeted opinion management. Through the professional application of behavioural psychological strategies, unprecedented techniques of propaganda and manipulation have become possible.[28] It is highly alarming to observe the penetrating power with which emotionally charged messages and headlines can be used to manipulate public opinion and general outrage behaviour, back and forth. Public opinion polls usually reflect the tenor of previous headlines, although the way such polls are asked often suggests the desired result in advance; when people are asked whether they would rather have compulsory masks at

---

27. See Anon, 'RS-Virus: Viele Kinder mit Infektionskrankheit im Klinikum Stuttgart' [RS virus: Many children with infectious diseases at Klinikum Stuttgart], *Stuttgarter Zeitung*, 29 November 2021; available at https://tinyurl.com/bddsvfk8 (accessed 27 June 2022).

28. Talk by Daniele Ganser, 'Propaganda – Wie unsere Gedanken und Gefühle gelenkt werden' [Propaganda – how our thoughts and feelings are guided], 12 April 2020; available at https://tinyurl.com/2p9dnuf9 (accessed 26 June 2020).

work or at home, over 90 per cent naturally say the workplace. If the headline then reads '90 per cent are in favour of compulsory masks at the workplace', this was not a genuine opinion poll but, rather, choreographed propaganda.[29]

The most effective and proven instrument for the abuse of power is the targeted operation with fears – fear of viruses, illness and death, of terrorists, Islamists, refugees, of job loss, social exclusion and social decline – all these latently existing fears can be used with the appropriate psychological finesse in a highly reliable way to specifically push through hidden, mostly business interests. Today, gigantic turnovers are generated with the cryptic promise of liberation from fear: insurance companies, armament companies, security technologies, e.g. cars like the SUVs that look like they're designed to win a war; but also the world's largest industrial sector, the health industry, isn't far behind in promising the allure of a fear-free world. They all promise health and safety not through peaceful and humane living conditions, but through 'products'. Many a senseless chemotherapy is sold as a 'last hope' – and at grotesquely high prices.

The most dangerous product of media psycho-techniques are the enemy images that have been produced in the run-up to most wars in order to divert attention from one's own aggressive motives. Former US President Jimmy Carter called the USA the most warlike nation in world history.[30] In its more than 240-year history, there have only been 16 years without war. This

29. See also Thomas Hardtmuth, 'Medienpsychologische Aspekte zur Corona-krise' [Media psychological aspects of the Corona crisis], in M. Glöckler & A. Neider (eds), *Corona – was uns die Pandemie lehren kann* [Corona – What the Pandemic Can Teach Us], Book on Demand, Stuttgart, 2022, pp. 223–42.
30. See Brett Wilkins, 'Jimmy Carter: die USA sind "die kriegerischste Nation der Weltgeschichte"' [Jimmy Carter: the US is 'the most belligerent nation in world history'], *Telepolis*, 21 April 2019; available at https://tinyurl.com/ycxvmc92 (accessed 26 June 2022).

self-proclaimed world power maintains military bases all over the world. Through elaborate secret service and 'intelligence' operations, the political and economic power elites (not the population) have destabilised numerous, mainly non-compliant countries and instigated so-called regime changes. The entire Arab Spring was fuelled by media propaganda techniques, and has left a trail of death and devastation in the old cultural countries of Syria, Iraq, Afghanistan and Libya. One corrupts, bullies, sanctions and destabilises until hatred and aggression escalate, and the outbreaks of violence thus provoked can then be used in public as a justifying argument for military intervention by the supposed 'peacemakers'.

In its history, the Russian nation, unlike the USA, has mostly been the victim of wars of aggression, and has been increasingly encircled by the gradual eastward expansion of NATO, in blatant contradiction to the promises made to Michael Gorbachev in the context of German reunification. This is in no way intended to legitimise the current Russian invasion of Ukraine; but for a proper assessment of the situation, the aforementioned facts are an important part of the overall picture. Instead, as we write (Spring 2022), the mainstream media's drumbeat of hostility against Russia is being beaten at a suspiciously loud volume, thus preventing peaceful co-operation with Germany, as it has been repeatedly offered by the Russian side over the last 30 years, but which the USA has corrupted with all its might as a 'nightmare',[31] for a long time to come. According to George Friedman, the fusion of Russian raw material wealth with German know-how represents the greatest threat to the American claim to world power leadership, and must be avoided at all costs.

---

31. See the statement by the Startfor think-tank founder and CEO and expert on US foreign policy, George Friedman, at the Chicago Council on Global Affairs; Friedman, 'Europe: Destined for Conflict?, YouTube, 4 February 2015; available at https://tinyurl.com/2p8tx8bt (accessed 26 June 2022).

The 'evil' Russian currently seems to be taking the place of the 'uninoculated' as a newly revived and eagerly staged enemy image in the media. They are shunned and mobbed, Russian artists are no longer engaged, business relations are terminated, athletes are ostracised, etc., as if anything useful could be achieved by this, except that aggression and hatred are further fuelled. As Albert Einstein almost certainly said, trying to end war by the same means that created it has never worked historically.

We are leaving the much-vaunted 'freedom of the press' behind us by leaps and bounds. Since the Corona crisis, critical journalism, which is essential for any healthy democracy, has increasingly given way to a uniform propaganda apparatus that is mainly geared towards alarmism, fear-mongering and agitation. It has to be said resoundingly: the commercial mass media, with their violence-glorifying sensationalism, have contributed significantly to the brutalisation and decultivation of society in recent years. When one's own ideas, and thus one's cultural identity and self-respect, dwindle, one needs images of the enemy, one needs the 'bad guys' to make oneself look 'good' – an age-old ritual of compensatory self-appreciation. Once again, people are allowed to defame and denounce without restraint, 70 years of German peace diplomacy are swept away by a new euphoria for rearmament, fundamental rights are thrown overboard at will, critical voices on the subject of coronary heart disease are not even heard, but immediately acknowledged with expulsion, as was recently the case with a health insurance company boss who had finally demanded a transparent explanation of vaccination damage.

Growing poverty and famine worldwide, social conflicts, broken relationships, waves of bankruptcies, fear, unemployment, ruined livelihoods, loneliness, psychological disorders amongst children and young people on an alarming scale – all this is chalked up as 'unavoidable collateral damage' in the (actually pointless) fight against a virus, and is mentioned only marginally as a footnote in the reporting. The fact that the damage caused by the political measures now far exceeds the virus problem per se is barely mentioned, let alone addressed. Instead of voicing criticism where it belongs, the media outrage exhausts itself in shallow sentimentality. With such embarrassing slogans as 'Vaccination is love' on posters, T-shirts and stickers, no real enlightenment can be achieved.

It is downright shameful how, meanwhile, politics has allowed itself to be degraded to the dutiful vicarious agent of economic elites and their lobbyists, who have obviously become megalomaniacs.[32] And even more alarming is the failure of journalism, which has sacrificed its actual profession of critical questioning to what amounts to a soporific conformism. Instead of clearly naming the really urgent problems of this world and calling for co-operation in solidarity, the recognisably bought mainstream journals keep serving new business models driven by profit mania, for which the crises of this world can be instrumentalised again and again.

Due to the constant propaganda, diagnosable anxiety disorders are increasing at an alarming rate; they are always an indicator of an unhealthy society. Fear not only weakens our clear and independent thinking, but also our physical and psychological immune functions in the long term. Immunisation against manip-

32. See the informative interview with the former German Health Minister Horst Seehofer in which he unmistakably expresses the 'last word' of the pharmaceutical lobby and the powerlessness of politics in important decisions; available at https://tinyurl.com/2p9dvzr2(accessed 27 June 2022). Part of this interview is included in the TV programme 'Frontal 21', which in 2008 investigated the power of the Pharma industry on politics; available at https://tinyurl.com/2p8prp5e (accessed June 2022).

ulation and propaganda is today the most important instrument for defending a humane society. (See also Hardtmuth, 2022.)

The authoritarian nature of modern science

Another key aspect of appropriately contextualising our conversation about modern medical science is to consider the place of science more generally in modern culture. When we first started reading about the philosophy of science some decades ago, it was *de rigueur* that *true* science can only thrive in a milieu of freedom and the open-minded and respectful discussion of contested viewpoints. Books with titles like *Conjectures and Refutations* (Popper) and *Science in a Free Society* (Feyerabend) said it all.[33] As William Blake wrote all those years ago, 'Without contraries is no progression'.

What different times we live in today! The likes of philosophers of science Karl Popper and Paul Feyerabend must be turning in their graves. In practice, science has almost certainly never achieved the truly radical openness to which the likes of Feyerabend and Popper idealistically aspired – but it is difficult to imagine a science more contaminated and compromised than what we've witnessed over the past two years during the Corona crisis. Certainly, the importance of a deep engagement with the *sociology* of science has never been more important than it is today.

Science has been characterised as a power structure that enforces its authority and punishes dissenters[34] – a view that immediately takes us into what is highly complex territory. We

33. See Popper, 1963, and Feyerabend, 1978.
34. As well as many recent discussions of this question in the non-mainstream media, a very good academic discussion of this issue in its many complexities can be found in Brian Martin (ed.), *Confronting the Experts*, State University of New York Press, Albany, NY, 1996. See also Brian Martin, 'Experts, establishments and learning from struggle', *AHPb Magazine for Self & Society*, 7 (Summer), 2021; available at https://tinyurl.com/4a97t4v2 (accessed 27 June 2022).

certainly would see science (or *any* human institution, come to that) as entailing power structures in which both conscious and unconscious power issues are at play. Notice that this doesn't mean that we need to claim that *all* the 'output' of the natural sciences is therefore necessarily affected, or tainted, by virtue of these power structures and issues. Rather, all we would want to claim is that we can't ignore such power issues when making assessments about the legitimacy of science, and its manifold practices and outputs.[35]

There can certainly be no doubt that dissenters from mainstream scientific orthodoxy are sometimes punished and/or silenced; but we don't want, or need, to claim that this is some kind of *universal* characteristic of science – merely a feature of what we call 'captured science'. It is always an empirical question as to whether power hierarchies are having an undue influence on scientific knowledge, or whether dissent is being silenced in an unwarranted way. Every such case or claim needs to be investigated on its own particular merits, as a unique instance.

The distinction between science and scient*ism* can be a useful one.[36] 'Scientism' is akin to a label that denotes an attitude and *an orientation*, and not a descriptor that can be deployed in making an empirical assessment of whether a given piece of

35. For an extended conversation of these issues, see Ian Kidd and Richard House, 'The Long Interview: "We're all Feyerabendians now!": Where science and society meet – the contemporary relevance of Paul K. Feyerabend, 1924–94', *AHPb Magazine for Self & Society*, 6 (Winter), 2021; available at https://tinyurl.com/bdh4hus4 (accessed 27 June 2022).
36. See, for example, Tom Sorell, *Scientism: Philosophy and the Infatuation with Science*, Routledge, London, 1991; Ian J. Kidd, 'Reawakening to wonder: Wittgenstein, Feyerabend, and scientism', in J. Beale & I.J. Kidd (eds), *Wittgenstein and Scientism,* Routledge, Abingdon, 2017, pp. 101–15; and Ian J. Kidd, 'Feyerabend, science, and scientism', in K. Bschir & J. Shaw (eds), *Interpreting Feyerabend: Critical Essays*, Cambridge University Press, Cambridge, 2021, pp. 172–90.

science is of a reliable standard. This means that scientists who could justifiably be labelled as 'scientistic' will sometimes do good science, just as those who avowedly eschew 'scientism' are quite capable of doing bad science! So in at least some circles, the term 'scientistic' has become something of a lazy name-calling exercise that can unhelpfully close down any further thinking, and which needs far more thinking through than its casual name-calling deployment typically allows for.

So, 'scientism' *might* sometimes be an accurate label for describing both some of the champions of modern medical science, and also some of its output; but the quality and legitimacy of medical-scientific output is independent of whether or not it, or its researchers, can be labelled 'scientistic'. For the latter, we need to get into the (possibly far more interesting) territory of what distinguishes 'good' from 'bad' science, and what shared and accepted criteria we can invoke to make that demarcation. We might well be entering into a relativistic terrain here! Scientists whose work is labelled as 'pseudo-science' by mainstream scientists will themselves often label mainstream science as being 'pseudo-science'! – the case of complementary and alternative medicine being a case in point.[37]

Any discussion of science must also address the question of materialism, and the metaphysical assumptions that accompany scientific work that (implicitly or otherwise) assumes materialism to be true and a coherent world-view. But if the work that fundamentally challenges materialism developed by people like philosopher Howard Robinson, spiritual scientist Rudolf Steiner, transpersonal psychologist Charles Tart and others (to

---

37. For an interesting discussion in relation to Feyerabend's and Popper's philosophies of science, see Ian J. Kidd, 'A pluralist challenge to "integrative medicine": Feyerabend and Popper on the cognitive value of alternative medicine' (Kidd, 2013).

take just a few examples) has anything in it,[38] then to assume that scientific investigation that axiomatically assumes materialism to be true is unproblematic and not open to challenge *on its own metaphysical terms* is – ironically – a very unscientific move to make.

It would be impossible to deny that there exist many examples of what is patently invalid 'anti-science denialism'. Yet contrary to mainstream narratives, it doesn't necessarily follow from this that *anyone* who challenges 'the science' (in whatever way) from a position of not being formally trained in the science under consideration is necessarily wrong or ill-informed. In their path-breaking book, subtitled *Why Everything You Thought You Knew about Medicine is Wrong*, Dawn Lester and David Parker make this latter point very convincingly (Lester & Parker, 2019). This is where engaging open-mindedly with philosophy and metaphysical presuppositions in relation to the practice of science comes in. The case of the Covid-19 injection treatments is a case in point. Something that can be construed as a 'success' at one (narrow) level of analysis ('the vaccine is safe and effective...') could easily become a disaster at another level of analysis.

Our view is that the deployment of 'the science' by the government-approved scientists and experts during the current Corona crisis has been extraordinary to behold, with simplistically positivistic and contestable claims cherry-picked to suit a seem-

38. See, for example, Howard Robinson, *Matter and Sense: A Critique of Contemporary Materialism*, Cambridge University Press, Cambridge, 1982; Rudolf Steiner, *Materialism and the Task of Anthroposophy*, Anthroposophic Press, Hudson, NY, 1987; Charles T. Tart, *The End of Materialism: How Evidence of the Paranormal is Bringing Science and Spirit Together*, New Harbinger, Oakland, Calif., 2009. See also Eric C. Martin, 'Late Feyerabend on materialism, mysticism, and religion', *Studies in History and Philosophy of Science*, Part A, 57 (June), 2016, pp. 129–36.

ingly pre-decided narrative not being subjected to any analysis or critique in the mainstream media because all dissenting *scientific* voices challenging the mainstream narrative have effectively been silenced. In an age of flagrant propagandising, like many others we wonder how citizens might be able to have easy access to all of the information needed from reputable sources in order to make empirical (scientific) assessments of such contested, literally life-changing issues.

The late aforementioned philosopher of science Paul K. Feyerabend was emphatic that it is an arrogant and unwarranted (not to mention incoherent) move for mainstream science to reject out of hand, and by definitional fiat, practices like homeopathy and astrology merely because they say so, from their materialistic metaphysical position that they just assume to be true.[39] Such hegemonic moves by mainstream science are, alas, all too common – for example, by mainstream medical science against complementary and alternative medicine, which, incredibly, even includes campaigns to make the practising of homeopathy and alternative medicine *illegal*. The practice of anthroposophical medicine is illegal in Quebec, for example.

Nearly half a century ago, Paul Feyerabend gave a prophetic lecture at the University of Sussex on the authoritarian tendencies of modern science[40] – and what he described then could hardly have more prescience than it does today. For Feyerabend, 'The excellence of science is assumed, it is not argued for'; and he makes a strong early case for science having be-

39. See, for example, Ian J. Kidd, 'Why did Feyerabend defend astrology? Integrity, virtue, and the authority of science', *Social Epistemology*, 30, 2016, pp. 464–82.
40. See Feyerabend's article, 'How to defend society against science', in *Radical Philosophy* 11, 1975, pp. 3–8. See also his books *Science in a Free Society* (Feyerabend, 1978), and *The Tyranny of Science*, (Feyerabend, 2011).

come The New Religion in modern culture. Thus,

> Scientists... act like the defenders of the One and Only
> Roman Catholic Church acted before them: Church doctrine
> is true, everything else is Pagan nonsense.... In society at
> large the judgement of the scientist is received with the same
> reverence as the judgement of bishops and cardinals was
> accepted not too long ago... [online]

If Feyerabend were alive today he would surely be arguing that, far from being the objective practice that it claims to be, 'the science' informing and underpinning the current putsch to vaccinate the world with an experimental, emergency-clearance medical procedure is bogus, disingenuous, and hopelessly compromised by infusions and abuses of institutional power, quasi-authoritarian 'regimes of truth' and vested financial interests. Notice that we have no need to invoke or deploy 'conspiracy theory' narratives to make this case – for as will be clear in the conversation that forms the core of this book, it can be convincingly made simply by virtue of turning the cannons and truth-aspirations of modern mainstream science against itself, and exposing the hopelessly incoherent 'scientific' case that is being made to support mass Covid-19 vaccination.

Yet we do need to ask to what extent there *might* conceivably be a genuine conspiracy occurring around mass Covid-19 vaccination – or whether the unfolding psychodrama has far more to do with the internal processes of scientific (human) institutions in the face of uncontainable anxiety and fear, with a kind of mass unconscious hysteria having taken hold.[41] How else might we account for the current extraordinary collapse of 'science' into what is little more than ideological propaganda?

41. For a very good, psychoanalytically informed discussion of what the terms 'mass formation', see Mattias Desmet, *The Psychology of Totalitarianism*, Chelsea Green Publishing, White River Junction, Vermont, 2022 – especially Part I, 'Science and Its Psychological Effects'.

We can turn to Feyerabend for some possible answers to these urgent questions.

It was in 1974 that Feyerabend gave his talk at the University of Sussex, provocatively titled 'How to defend society against science'. In that lecture, he said:

> I want to defend society and its inhabitants from all ideologies, science included. There is nothing inherent in science... that makes it essentially liberating.... *Science has now become as oppressive as the ideologies it had once to fight....* Heretics in science are still made to suffer from the most severe sanctions this relatively tolerant civilization has to offer.... Science has become rigid, [and] *it has ceased to be an instrument of change and liberation.... Modern science... inhibits freedom of thought....*
>
> The competence... and the successes of science are vastly exaggerated.... The progress of... good science depends on novel ideas and on intellectual freedom.... Most scientists today are devoid of ideas, full of fear, intent on producing some paltry result so that they can add to the flood of inane papers that now constitutes 'scientific progress' in many areas. (our added italics) [online]

These criticisms are searing and uncompromising – yet many of the tendencies we can observe in science in the Corona era are observable in these observations from nearly half a century ago. Perhaps it should come as no surprise that in an age of acute, uncontainable anxiety, such formerly nascent authoritarian tendencies should come to prominence.[42]

Several years after his 1974 talk, Feyerabend wrote his most controversial book – *Science in a Free Society*. It is here that Feyerabend starts actually naming the incipient authoritarianism of the modern scientific attitude and its associated practices. For

---

42. See Desmet, ibid.

Feyerabend, rather than being a liberator of thought as it has long claimed, scientific rationality today acts as a form of suppression, often inhibiting and silencing any rivals to its narrowly positivist, dogmatic worldview, and imposing a set of doctrines and procedures administered and institutionalised by 'experts' that effectively stifle most if not all criticism.[43] Sound familiar?... He goes as far as to claim that authoritarian, out-of-control scientific rationalism threatens democracy itself by the way in which what he calls 'an unholy alliance of science, rationalism and capitalism', an 'intellectual fascism', crushes all opposition to its hegemony.

In stark contrast, Feyerabend champions a society of free interchange in which science is but one of many voices, and he thus advocates a fundamental reassessment of the role of science in modern culture. For Feyerabend, freedom is the ultimate human value, and he is challenging a core Enlightenment premise – namely, that intellectual and societal progress can only be achieved through the control of reason with the help of science.

Feyerabend insists that non-scientific alternatives may sometimes work as well, or even better, than mainstream scientific procedures. We read that 'Man once possessed complex knowledge concerning his place in nature, [but this] knowledge has been replaced by abstract theories he does not understand and *must take on trust from experts*' (our italics). And with particular relevance to the Covid-19 era, we read that '[scientific] unanimity is the result of shared prejudices: positions are taken without detailed examination of the matter under review... A unanimity that rests on "internal" considerations alone often turns out to be mistaken.'

Feyerabend also refers to 'the incompetence of scientific medicine as a whole', referring to the 'fantastic incompetence of

43. See Martin, note 34.

modern scientific medicine remain[ing] hidden from the public'. He notes that 'Our ancestors and "primitive" contemporaries had highly developed... medical theories and biological doctrines that are often more adequate and have better results than their Western competitors and describe phenomena not accessible to an "objective" laboratory approach....'. Moreover, 'Comprehensive mistakes involving the "basic ideology" of the field can be often revealed only by outsiders or by scientists with an unusual personal history'.

Feyerabend also addresses the interpenetration of science with business and financial interests. He writes, 'an independent science has long ago been replaced by the business science which lives off society and strengthens its totalitarian tendencies' – with 'many parts of science now [becoming] businesses when the aim is no longer to find truth... but to keep the money coming in'. And today, 'science prevails not because of its comparative merits, but because the show has been rigged in its favour.... The superiority of science is not the result of research, or argument, it is the result of political, institutional, and even military pressures.'

Finally, in a passage that has an eerie resonance with science in the era of Corona, we read of the 'narcissistic chauvinism' of science, and that

> scientists have now the power to impose their ideology on almost everyone... – with a large part of the general public [being] hypnotized by science... . [They] are parasites of the mind and they will continue in their path until democracy puts them in their place...[with] the technological approach with its inbuilt distrust of nature, its conceited belief in the excellence of science, and its determination to remake man and nature in its own image.

And in what is an extraordinarily prophetic reference, we read that 'killing in the scientific manner is legal while healing in the non-scientific manner is outlawed'.

This extended critical discussion of the place of science in contemporary society provides a lengthy but necessary backdrop to the conversation that forms the heart of this book.

*****

This introduction has attempted to contextualise the in-depth conversation that follows about the state of modern biomedicine and the urgent need for a new paradigm of health, well-being and healing.

The Dialogue

Richard House [RH]: Thomas, thank you so much for agreeing to this interview; it's an honour for me to be able to have a conversation with someone as knowledgeable as you on these crucial issues. May I begin by asking you to share something of your own professional journey, and at what point in your unfolding career you realised that immunity is such a key issue in relation to health and illness?

Thomas Hardtmuth [TH]: Already in the course of my medical studies I was dealing with psychosomatic medicine, and especially with the anthroposophically oriented healing arts. Through numerous working groups and 30 years of practical experience as a doctor, I became more and more aware that autonomy issues play a central role in human health. 'Autonomy' is understood in the salutogenic sense as *the ability to self-regulate and thus experience self-efficacy in one's own life*.

During my ten years as a lecturer for health sciences and social medicine at the Dual University of Baden-Württemberg, I chose this autonomy theme as the guiding principle for my lectures. Some of my publications on contemporary diseases, such as cancer, depression and dementia, also dealt with this topic (Hardtmuth, 2011). In 2020 a book, *Perspektiven einer Biologie der Freiheit* (Perspectives of a Biology of Freedom) was published (edited by Bernd Rosslenbroich, an evolutionary biologist), where I summarised my experiences in this area under the title 'Autonomy and health' (Hardtmuth, 2020a).

What autonomy consists in on the spiritual-cultural level is what we call 'resilience' in the soul realm, and at the biological level these are the immune functions. All three levels cannot be separated: it is always the human ego-forces that are visible in differing ways on the three different levels.

RH: So as I understand it, Thomas, we have *self-regulation* at the spiritual-cultural level; *resilience* in terms of mental health; and *immunity* at the biological level; and taken together, this is an *holistic* human phenomenon that cannot be disaggregated into autonomous self-contained parts. Does it follow from this that in terms of effective 'medical' treatment informed by an all-encompassing scientific approach, it is not appropriate to treat just one of these three levels without addressing the other two levels as well? So that in the case of immunity, for example, to 'treat' it merely through a 'medical-model' approach (like vaccination) without addressing the other two levels cannot but be, at best, a partial approach – and at worst, could be a woefully inadequate (or even *iatrogenic*) treatment.[44]

I am also struck by how what, in some circles, is called the 'Victimhood Archetype' (e.g. Hall, 1993) plays into the picture you've so usefully painted here. Victimhood is the very opposite of what you term 'self-efficacy' and 'self-regulation': the core metaphysical belief which the 'victimhood mentality' assumes is that we inhabit a deterministic universe in which hu-

44. Iatrogenesis (from which term the adjective 'iatrogenic' derives) is the causation of a disease, a harmful complication, or other ill-effect by any medical activity, including diagnosis, intervention, error or negligence; in other words, when medical treatment itself does harm. See, for example, Sharpe & Faden, 1998. It has been estimated in peer-reviewed research that about 330,000 patients a year die from prescription drugs in the USA and Europe, with 80 million patients suffering 'side-effects' of pains, discomforts, dysfunctions etc. Source: Light, 2014; see also Light et al., 2013.

man beings (and their symptoms) are *caused* (e.g. by our genes) – and that we are therefore the victims of whatever those external causes might be.

It seems to me that the practice of vaccination is a paradigm-case of a medical treatment that is underpinned by such a 'victimhood' mentality – that is, the accompanying, self-justifying narrative says that our illness is 'caused' by a virus, so all we need to do in this mechanistic universe is to eliminate, neutralise or control the cause (i.e. the virus) – for example, via a vaccine – and then, ipso facto, we will be healthy again. How seductively simple! – and no need to take responsibility for anything other than rolling up our sleeve to get the jab! (In passing, I've always been very suspicious of such simplistic causal, 'positivistic' thinking; and I just read in another of your publications about science's 'out-of-date bio-mechanistic understanding of nature and the human being', which assumes an isolated chain of causes but seems unable (or unwilling) to grasp the *systemic* relationships that surely need to inform any full understanding of micro-organisms. How I agree with that!)

In stark contrast, a *self-efficacy* approach to the human being clearly requires that we address the other levels you refer to – which I assume has as a core precept that we take full responsibility for our own health and well-being – and all that this entails. I had no idea this interview was going to begin in this manner! – but do my musings make any sense to you in relation to your own way of understanding these questions? And perhaps in the process of your reply, you could say something about the worldview entailed by psychosomatic medicine[45] and the anthroposophically oriented healing arts – and how their

45. Psychosomatic medicine is an interdisciplinary medical field exploring the relationships among social, psychological and behavioural factors on bodily processes and quality of life in humans and animals.

whole approach to medicine differs from the mainstream 'medical model'.

TH: I will try and address the individual points that you raise. Of course we cannot consider the three levels of autonomy in isolation. Medicine in the future must be an integrated form of medicine that is not solely based on biological mechanisms, but is broadened to include, for example, the biopsychosocial model developed by the American psychiatrist George L. Engel (1977), and included long before that in the principles underpinning anthroposophic medicine. This approach to medicine thinks in terms of 'forces' – in the anthroposophical context we speak of 'etheric medicine' – which come to expression in different ways on the physiological, psychological and mental levels,[46] but nonetheless originate from the same source – namely, from our individuality.

There is far more to strengthening the immune system than giving biotechnological stimulation with a vaccine. The significance of vaccines in the control of infectious disease epidemics is vastly overrated because in the industrialised world, the influence of psychosocial factors on human health is deliberately excluded. There are no profits to be made with salutogenesis.[47] This is the fundamental error in our health system – namely, that money can be made from illness, and that a sick society offers a profitable market place. It was the introduction of the all-consuming neoliberal economic logic of the 1980s that

---

46. *Psychological* problems are commonly perceived to be a result of environmental factors or social circumstances, thus placing responsibility on external factors typically beyond the person's control. *Mental* problems are perceived to be caused by individual 'weakness' or genetic faults – internal factors that can potentially be controlled.

47. The term 'salutogenesis' refers to the origins of health, focusing on factors that support human health and well-being, rather than on factors that cause disease (pathogenesis).

transformed the healthcare system into a market place. This also turned pandemics into a highly lucrative business model that has been kept well-oiled by ever-more brazen attempts at ramping up fear. Giovanni Maio, the well-known professor of ethics at the University of Freiburg, had expressly warned of this development in his books (for example in *Geschäftsmodell Gesundheit – wie der Markt die Heilkunst abschafft* (e.g. Hontschik & Maio, 2014).

Now to the concept of sacrifice. We must of course distinguish between the sacrifice I make consciously in response to a situation, out of dedication or love etc., i.e. what I do out of *freedom*; and the sacrificial role that plays out unconsciously as a result of conditioning and education, or through passivity and dependency. In the first case, my 'I' is fully present, and I engage with the issues myself; in the second case, the problems control me, and I play catch-up with them. This defensive 'archetype of victimhood' is, as you describe, being massively stimulated by the Corona propaganda.

Since we are human, there are of course many intermediate forms, too. The person who founded the concept of salutogenesis, Aaron Antonovsky, said that health is not a passive condition but *a permanently active process* in which we continually seek to overcome and learn from the tendencies that make us ill. He spoke of a health–illness continuum which, as human beings, we are continually moving through. We also live in an ongoing tension between autonomy and heteronomy, i.e. between self-determination and being determined from outside. The importance of autonomy for health should not be seen as an absolute, since it gives rise to the stand-alone illusion and egocentric focus that is so widespread today, and the many associated conditions of loneliness, especially within the growing singleton culture of big cities. We are 'I' beings *and*, simultaneously, social beings. Heteronomy in this context has not only pathogenetic significance; it also embraces belonging, participating, sacrificing, forgetting oneself, recognising oneself in the other. We *share* our lives with each other. The fact that we can identify ourselves with the 'I' of the other person provides the greatest incentive for the evolution of a common, human culture.

But pathology arises on all three levels of autonomy when the positive self-image of a human being and, with it, authenticity and self-efficacy (we can also say *self-empowerment*), are completely and permanently lost. A kind of alien life then begins to emancipate itself in the person. On the biological level, it is the viruses and bacteria that take on a life of their own and develop as infectious diseases. With cancerous growth there is also a form of 'alien autonomy' that spreads through the organism. On the soul level, the hidden self makes itself felt through anxiety, self-harm and compulsive behaviour, through to psychotic events in which the human being is totally dominated by this alien element.

I completely agree with your perception that the metaphysical conviction of a deterministic universe is the medium for growing the bio-mechanistic ideology which has such an influence on today's medicine. It has no real concept of the ego and the latter's concrete physiological activity. In discussions about infection, the focus is placed exclusively on exposure, and too little attention is given to constitution and disposition.

Determinism is unable to develop a concept of freedom, nor of health, because it is imprisoned in a one-dimensional, physical pattern of causal thinking which can only explain things in terms of past conditions. The neurobiological determinism which swept through the media a few years ago with the message 'Not I but the brain decides' was, for me, just a foretaste of its escalation today in the Corona crisis – the last gasp of a long decadent materialistic dogma – with a massive attack on the human 'I' and its freedom. *Using the sophisticated psychological techniques of ongoing media propaganda, a climate of fear and confusion was created whose long-term effects are the very opposite of the health it was supposedly intended to support.*

Chronic fear and powerlessness, helplessness and social isolation are anti-ego forces, and therefore the most effective killers of immunity that we know of. This global pandemic of fear, with all its martial measures, will be shown to have caused far more suffering and death that the virus itself; and in any case, contemporary knowledge shows that the paradigm of a single virus causing a specific illness is increasingly questionable.

RH: Thank you for this wonderfully incisive answer, Thomas; it puts into clear persective many if not most of the concerns that have motivated us to dive deeply into this conversation. There are several lines I'd like to pursue from your answer, but first, I have not before come across Giovanni's Maio's fascinating-sounding book *Business Model of Health – How the Market is Abolishing the Art of Healing*: rarely can one book title have conveyed so much in so few words! (Maio, 2014)

I'm wondering whether one could also stretch this even further, to say that 'the market' also '"abolishes" *true* science', as well – in that when it is the money-making profit motive that drives medicine and medical activity, then what succeeds in making the *most* money (i.e. profit maximisation) is almost bound to trump and prevail over everything else – and that includes an honest, genuinely open-minded attitude and approach to scientific theory and praxis – with the latter being one of the first casualties of 'business-model health'. Or put differently, perhaps the great danger here is that 'the science' will be constructed in the image of the market, and will then *necessarily* be distorted, and thus diverted from what should be a fearless adherence to the best of scientific praxis, wherever it might lead. And furthermore, all of the actors involved in this system, who have a vested interest in the fruits that this model produces, will be motivated to align themselves with this distorted model of 'science', rather than with truly authentic science.

Does what I'm saying here make sense to you? I'd really welcome your thoughts on and insights into this phenomenon; and do you know of anyone (yourself included!) who has written at length on how *science itself* has been distorted because of its colonisation by neoliberal free-market ideology?

TH: Richard, what you are suggesting here puts the finger directly into the wound of a sick medicine! Good science proves itself primarily in the questions it asks, not so much in the answers it gives. There is often much more spirit and intelligence in a good question than in the answers; it is the wise question, which presupposes a free spirit, which opens up the space for creative and innovative research. Today, we are miles away from this Humboldtian ideal of education and science.[48] The horizon within which current medical research takes place is so narrow that it is increasingly becoming a dead end. The guidelines of the industrial-pharmacological complex determine not

---

48. Wilhelm von Humboldt (1767–1835) was a Prussian philosopher, linguist, government functionary and diplomat, particularly remembered as a linguist who made important contributions to the philosophy of language, ethnolinguistics and to the theory and practice of education. He envisioned education as a means of realising individual possibility rather than a way of drilling traditional ideas into young people. He was the architect of the Humboldtian education ideal, used in Prussia as a model for its public education system.

only what is researched, but – and this is the real evil – what is *not* researched.

Let me give you an example. In the case of metastasised cancer, palliative chemotherapies are carried out today, which, for example, in the case of lung cancer are sold as a 'last chance' and achieve a statistical prolongation of life of 3–4 weeks – but in reality, they essentially amount to a prolongation of dying. Such mostly pointless therapy regimes cost between 100,000 and 150,000 euros per treatment, and researchers no longer even ask about fundamentally alternative concepts. Instead, they only ever compare chemotherapy A with chemotherapy B, and do not even notice how they've been spinning in circles for decades on the shackle of this one-dimensional battle strategy of aggressive cell elimination.

Individualised therapy approaches of an integral medicine, which work with all three autonomy levels mentioned earlier, certainly have a far better outcome. But this cannot be 'proven' because the primacy of statistics as the sole criterion of evidence forces us to use standard therapies that presuppose a 'standard' patient – which does not exist in reality. The methodological constraints of medical research categorically do not, therefore, take into account the influence of autonomy factors on the healing process! The individual simply does not exist in this science. This is the fundamental systemic error in established medical thinking that I have been talking about. The problem is not only that the biographical-psychosocial, especially the chronic stress factors, are given far too little consideration, but also that most of the modern findings of psychoneuroimmunology, genome research and epigenetics[49] have been slept through, which simply show what a decisive influence self-regulation processes

49. 'Epigenetics' refers to the study of how human behaviours and environment can cause changes that affect the way our genes work.

have right down to the genes.

I'll give one example here. Katharina Domschke from the University Clinic in Freiburg was able to show that long-term depression and anxiety, which we now know are often the initial symptoms of chronic diseases, are associated with epigenetic changes that can be reversed after just four weeks of psychotherapy. One could cite numerous other examples. In a recent study at the University of Ulm (Clemens et al., 2018), people who had been sexually abused or had been subjected to other experiences of violence in childhood were observed over a long period of time. Among numerous other disease risks, these people had a six-fold (!) increased risk of carcinoma because their entire stress biology was in a kind of permanent state of alert. Here, targeted, preventive salutogenetic and psychotherapeutic measures would be far more sensible (and cost-effective) than just running after the disease process with toxic and grotesquely expensive chemotherapies.

The latest studies regarding human genome sequencing show more and more clearly how highly individual the human organism is also on the biological level. Our unique intestinal microbiome alone leads to a highly individual metabolisation of medicines, so that standardised treatment approaches alone are becoming increasingly questionable. Every person develops a personal relationship with a medicine – this is not a metaphor, but reality! Our immune system develops in a way that is complementary to the gut microbiome and carries an equally individual signature.

Unfortunately, as has to be said so clearly, in recent decades the economic logic of profit maximisation has increasingly become the leading motive of medical research. The spread of fear of disease and death inevitably becomes a lucrative marketing concept, as can easily be observed today.

Christian Kreiß, an economist at Aalen University, has written a very informative book that is well worth reading about the increasing, disastrous fusion of economics and medicine: *Gekaufte Forschung – Wissenschaft im Dienst der Konzerne* (Kreiss, 2015) (in translation, Purchased Research – Science in the Service of the Corporations).

RH: A wonderfully rich answer again, Thomas. I think this point is absolutely key – that 'Good science proves itself primarily in the questions it asks, not so much in the answers it gives'. And the *presuppositions* one holds about reality and the cosmos will be a very major influence on the questions one is able to ask, and even conceive of (remember Einstein sitting on that tram in Zurich and imagining that now legendary thought-experiment!...). So, for example, if one assumes *at the outset* that a virus is 'pathogenic' and has to be destroyed in an all-out 'war' by all available technological means (what you evocatively refer to as a 'one-dimensional battle strategy of aggressive cell elimination'), then of course the 'answers' one is able to reach will be severely constrained by one's initial, assumed worldview. And woe betide us all if the initial assumptions on which such a 'declaration of war on nature' are based are just plain wrong! Not least, we end up, as you say, with '... the horizon within which current medical research takes place [being] so narrow that it is increasingly becoming a dead end' (and 'dead' not just in a metaphorical sense, perhaps).

Earlier, you touched on this whole question of fallacious assumptions leading to false, and possibly catastrophic consequences, when you said:

> Chronic fear and powerlessness, helplessness and social isolation are... the most effective immune killers that we know.

This global fear pandemic with all the martial measures will cause far more suffering and death than the virus itself....
The paradigm of a single virus as the causative agent of a specific disease is becoming increasingly questionable due to the latest findings. (my italics)

Could you say more about this, and your latest understanding of the truest and best-available science around all this? (as opposed to Big Pharma's narrow medical-research horizon).

Relatedly, perhaps, you also recently wrote to me in personal correspondence that 'we have to talk more about a dynamic sphere, than about specific microbes. What we constantly absorb from the virosphere are quasi-biological "inspirations" that drive evolution forward – but not deterministically...'. This feels like the early intimations of a *genuinely new* scientific paradigm, Thomas; it would be very exciting if you could sketch out here what that new scientific paradigm might look like, and what it is in the old (Big Pharma) paradigm that needs replacing and transcending – for the sake of our healthy human future.

These are big questions, I know – but I also know that you are singularly well equipped to answer them. (I also realise that to articulate a new and convincing paradigm is one thing; but to actually *get* to and implement it, in the teeth of the massive opposition it will no doubt face from the entrenched interests supporting the current flawed paradigm, is quite another question – and perhaps more of a sociological, political and democratic question; but that's perhaps for another conversation.)

TH: The paradigm of the specific aetiology[50] of infectious diseases – one pathogen, one disease, one therapy – was established

---

50. 'Aetiology' refers to the study of the cause, set of causes or manner of causation of a disease or condition.

in the second half of the nineteenth century by Robert Koch and Louis Pasteur. The discovery of specific micro-organisms identified in the context of tuberculosis, anthrax, diphtheria, etc. was a scientific sensation at the time, which found rapid and high acceptance in society because the new 'enemy image' of bacteria resonated with a simple traditional pattern of thought; in a spirit of time shaped by militarism, the 'declaration of war against bacteria' provided a strategy that was immediately obvious to everyone. In his famous lecture on bacteriological research on 4 August 1890 to hundreds of doctors and scientists from all over the world at the Charité – a military hospital under the command of the General Staff – Robert Koch ended with the following words:

> And so let me conclude this lecture with the wish that the forces of the nations may measure themselves in this field of work and in war against the smallest but most dangerous enemies of the human race, and that in this struggle for the good of all mankind, one nation will always outstrip the other in its successes.

With this, a battle mentality, as already established by Darwinism, was also introduced into medicine; the disease of man was replaced by an animal model, which was linked to eradication fantasies; and this utopia, that viruses could be 'destroyed', has been deeply engraved in the thinking habits of people and, above all, of science right to the present day. A huge industry still lives based on the enemy-image of micro-organisms.

However, the findings of microbiome research in the last 10–15 years have increasingly confirmed what was already emphasised by the critics of the germ theory in the nineteenth century: 'Le microbe n'est rien, le terrain est tout' ('The germ is nothing, the terrain is everything'). Louis Pasteur is said to have confirmed this sentence of the French physician Antoine Béchamp on his death-bed (Hume, 2017/1923). Max von Pettenkofer, a Munich polymath and opponent of Koch, who is considered to be the founder of hygiene science, drank half a litre of a suspension with cholera bacteria in front of a large audience without falling ill from it, the aim being to demonstrate that microbes alone do not cause disease.

We now know that well over 90 per cent of all infectious diseases, such as tuberculosis, diphtheria, cholera and many more, have declined simply due to improvements in living conditions, long before the first vaccines and antibiotics were introduced (see Černič, 2018). At the beginning of the Industrial Revolution, most people in the cities lived in miserable conditions; small, dark, damp flats with mould and bad air, no adequate heating, with poverty, scarcity, stress, cold, miserable hygiene and the daily fear of survival; *these* were the main reasons for the epidemics, not the bacteria.

Today, modern microbiome research educates us to think in systems terms – not in antiquated, one-dimensional explanatory patterns, but in complex, living contexts. Anthroposophically speaking, we are in the age of the development of the consciousness-soul, and I have the feeling that the Corona crisis is like a last gasp of a reductionist-biomechanistic mind–soul culture that has become decadent. At the end of the Middle Ages, it was symptoms of decadence such as the Inquisition, the indulgence and relic trade that ushered in the end of the morbid, clerical power elites before the Enlightenment took hold. I see a similar phase today: the fear of viruses and witches has a similar psychological background, perhaps to exaggerate somewhat (but only somewhat!). The Enlightenment is indeed far from over!

You asked me about the new scientific understanding that

marks a broader horizon than that of Big Pharma. I would like to illustrate this with an example. In a study published in 2017 (Moustafa et al., 2017), virome analyses in the blood of 8,240 asymptomatic, healthy individuals showed 94 different virus species, with 19 species alone detectable in 42 per cent of the subjects. These included not only herpes and anelloviruses[51] but also various types of so-called cancer-causing viruses and other supposedly pathogenic species such as the AIDS pathogen HIV, hepatitis B and C viruses, polyoma and parvoviruses.[52] What does this mean?

If we consider that evolution on earth began with viruses, then it is hardly surprising that our entire organism is riddled with viruses. Viruses have been an integral part of all living things from the beginning! But they are not parasitic poisonous creatures – something which is still claimed and often assumed today. In the human genome, 46,000 retroviruses and about 1.5 million virus fragments have now been identified, i.e. the genomes of all living beings are basically made up of viruses! This is the most spectacular scientific discovery of the twenty-first century. Genetic evolution and biodiversity ultimately mean the incorporation of ever-new viruses.

Now you may understand from this why I am talking about a paradigm shift. We have to completely rethink this whole field, and form new, more realistic concepts. Viruses are not pathogens in a mono-causal sense. If, instead of a colourful variety of flowers, only dandelions grow on an over-fertilised meadow, then the dandelions are not pathogens, but a symptom of a sick

---

51. Anelloviruses are small, single-stranded circular DNA viruses. They are extremely diverse, and have not to date been associated with any disease. Strikingly, these small entities infect most probably the complete human population, and there are no convincing examples demonstrating viral clearance from infected individuals.

52. Polyoma and parvoviruses are animal viruses.

system. And it is similar with infectious diseases when individual micro-organisms, which are otherwise only present in reasonable numbers in a healthy mixed culture, appear pathologically as a monoculture.

Basically, we would have to write a pathology of monocultures, because in my opinion they are the central systemic health problem, not only in the biological and ecological sense, but also in the social, psychological and spiritual sense.

RH: I'm in awe at both the clarity and authority of this answer, Thomas, and also excitedly blown away by the content and implications of what you're saying here. For if what you're saying in the above is anything like right, and we also assume that the truth will 'out' eventually and be accepted by the 'kicking and screaming' mainstream, we could right now be in the middle of the kind of *scientific revolution* that philosopher Thomas Kuhn wrote about 60 years ago – and which is precisely why I wanted to engage in 'revolutionary' conversations such as this one.

Your point about pathological monocultures reminded of Vandana Shiva's excellent work on 'monocultures of the mind' (Shiva, 1993, p. 7) – where she writes, for example, that

> Monocultures first inhabit the mind. Then as a monoculture takes root, they have a characteristic relation to the world around them.... Monocultures of the mind generate models of production which *destroy diversity and legitimise that destruction as progress*, growth and improvement. ... *[This leads to] impoverished systems* both qualitatively and quantitatively. They are also highly unstable and non-sustainable systems not because they produce more, but because they control more. *The expansion of monocultures has more to do with politics and power than with enriching and enhancing systems.* (my italics)

I'm always fascinated when statements written in another context can have deep resonances in putatively unrelated fields! I think there exists a very rich and insightful vein of thinking here that could easily be applied to mainstream medical science and allopathic medicine, too. A book on *The Pathology of Monocultures* would indeed make a tremendous contribution!

Relatedly, it is fascinating to hear about some of the origins of this 'battle mentality' you speak of in relation to viruses and pathogens, and how it has become (often unconsciously) inscribed into the very 'psyche' (if I may use that term) of modern medical science. I think there is also a cultural story to be told about *patriarchy* here (e.g. Kashtan, 2017), and the way in which a fundamentally patriarchal world-view (again unconsciously) underpins so much medical science – and which is then 'acted out' (to use a psychoanalytic term) in ways that the protagonists and apologists for the status quo are completely unaware of, and which they then delude themselves to be 'objective science'! But that's another story and for another conversation, perhaps.

There are many directions in which I'd like to take our emerging dialogue, Thomas; but can I ask what you think are the main impediments to this 'revolution' happening. I'm speaking here of the forces – cultural, political-economic, egotistical-psychological, paradigmatic, bureaucratic-institutional, professional, spiritual… – that will be determined to retain, and even entrench still further, the mainstream status quo, and concomitantly, will attempt to rubbish and discredit any ideas, insights, new theories etc. that propose a worldview and medical ontology[53]

53.   The term 'ontology' refers to the branch of philosophy that studies concepts such as existence, being, becoming, and reality – or in short, theories of what exists. It includes the questions of how entities are grouped into basic categories and which of these entities exist on the most fundamental level.

that flatly contradict germ theory and many/most of the other *leitmotifs* of modern medical science. Another way of putting this might be: how, in the real, existing world of inherently conservative, system-reinforcing tendencies and vested interests, is much-needed change actually going to happen? And of course I don't underestimate what a complex and involved question this is!

TH: Richard, I have no illusions that the 'scientific revolution' of which we or Thomas S. Kuhn have spoken of will still take a few decades before what is now called 'systems science' – we could also call it 'the science of living connections' – begins to develop.

In addition to the Corona crisis, it will take some more painful mistakes and experiences before we free ourselves from the constraints of 'biomechanistic ideology', and find what the evolutionary biologist Wolfgang Schad[54] calls 'the peripheral view' (Schad, 2014). Today, we think from the point to the periphery, from the atom to the universe; we spend a huge amount of time and effort (for example, at the Cern nuclear research facility in Geneva) arriving at an understanding of cosmic laws, a universal formula deduced from the analysis of elementary particles. It is the same one-dimensional centrifugal way of thinking that thinks from virus to disease or pandemic. Of course, micro-organisms are *part* of the understanding of epidemics; but without an understanding of the immunological, psychosocial and ecological connections, we will not be able to develop a real concept of health, and new 'epidemics' (in the broadest sense) will always appear.

54. Evolutionary biologist Professor Wolfgang Schad worked for many years as a Waldorf school teacher and as a lecturer at the Waldorf Teacher's College in Stuttgart. He is an Emeritus Professor at the Institute for Evolutionary Biology, University of Witten-Herdecke, Germany, a position he held until his retirement in 2005.

A healthy science breathes between the centrifugal and centripetal movements of thought, from the whole to the detail and back again. The revolution will be that we no longer conceive of life as a property of matter, but as an ontologically irreducible level of reality. We cannot locate the living in space, we cannot say that life starts from a point; the living works where it establishes the connections of the points, which is an epistemologically fundamental act that must be realised in all concreteness; atomic power starts from the point, the living from the periphery. And it is precisely this living thinking that micro-organisms teach us in a very vivid way, as I have tried to describe in my new book on the microbiome (Hardtmuth, 2021).

I'll give you a practical example; we have to be very specific about this. One of the best-researched intestinal bacteria is *Escherichia coli*, which is found in the intestines of all mammals. Now, we must not think that this micro-organism has a stable identity like a bee, a rabbit or a human being. The strain genome of *E. coli* accounts for only 6 per cent, everything else is variable. For comparison: the genomes of Richard House and Thomas Hardtmuth are 99.9 per cent identical, those of humans and chimpanzees 98.7 per cent, and of mice and rats about 90 per cent. In other words, what we call '*E. coli*' are actually countless, genetically highly diverse organisms whose genome, and thus their properties, are highly plastic and flexible, depending on the situational context. They constantly change their genome, then, depending on the surrounding situation. This means that their existence and metabolism are not determined by themselves and their genome in the centre, but by the periphery. The ecosystem or the host organism decides how this bacterium behaves.

The large cattle farms in the USA produce gigantic amounts of dung, which are deposited into huge cesspools. This does not normally happen in nature, where millions of litres of faeces or trillions of *E. coli* bacteria come together in one place. Nature has to regulate this; the population dynamics of micro-organisms, i.e. which microbe occurs when, where, and in what numbers, are essentially regulated in ecosystems by viruses. In this case, this means that the 'monoculture' of coli bacteria must be attacked by a toxic virus so that the natural balance is restored. From the cesspools on the farms, these infected bacteria seep into the groundwater and, via contamination of the drinking water, lead to about 90,000 (sometimes fatal) EHEC[55] infections every year in the USA. So in order to understand this disease, we must not only look at the bacterium or the virus, but at the pathological ecosystem of cattle farms. The root cause is not the microbe as a point, but in the periphery of the interrelationships that we ourselves have caused.

This principle basically applies to all micro-organisms; that is, they are only to be understood as part of a larger whole – and therein will lie the paradigm shift we are speaking of. To think in a living way means to think anew every time, because the current contexts are always new.

You asked about the main obstacles that stand in the way of this new thinking. It is, as you also put it, always the old and cumbersome, patriarchal and authoritarian power structures – in the anthroposophical context we would speak of 'retarded spirits' – that have a paralysing effect on progress. Their only – albeit very effective – instrument of power is fear, as can easily be observed at the present time.

People who see the meaning of their existence only in the elitist

---

55. EHEC refers to *enterohaemorrhagic Escherichia coli*, a disease which causes severe diarrhoea with kidney failure.

exercise of power and in boundless wealth will always perish at some point from their own greatness and decadence, like the dinosaurs 60 million years ago; that is like a law of nature! Nature does not tolerate monocultures: its principle is that of *dynamic diversity* – at all levels! Everything imperial and totalitarian in history is characterised by the fact that it has perished – and mostly in a catastrophic scenario. Only rarely have the established power structures changed through self-reflection and insight.

What will always remain, on the other hand, is the creative human being. The most important thing we can do today is to teach children how to think in a living way! Educational institutions, especially Steiner Waldorf schools, would have to take the Corona crisis as an opportunity to teach the incredible dynamics and plasticity of microbial life on earth as the basis of an almost unlimited and diverse evolution, as opposed to implementing a deep mistrust of nature with the enemy-image of viruses we discussed earlier. This image of a creative universe creates in the souls of children the prerequisite for mobile, lively and innovative thinking.

We have to be aware that evolution, if we translate it into one week, has dealt only with micro-organisms from Monday to Saturday (3 billion years), and all 'visible' living beings have emerged on Sunday (600 million years). In India, the cow (their rumen contains around 20 kilos of bacteria) is revered as a sacred animal because it is a kind of representative of this metabolic wisdom on earth, which works from the periphery via the microbiosphere and keeps us all alive.

RH: I just read a chapter by another big thinker, David Ray Griffin, written well over three decades ago, in which he wrote:

the transition from the modern to a postmodern paradigm…
will allow the evidence of psychosomatic interaction to be
taken seriously in the science of medicine, leading to significant modifications in both research and practice….. [Post-
modern medicine will] bring personal causation back into
science, a development that will encourage the full recognition of individual differences, *even at the level of biochemistry*…. Postmodern medicine will overcome the alienating de-
personalization that has been the bane of modern medicine.
(Griffin, 1988, p. 161, my italics)

So although siren voices raised against monocultural biomedical science have been around for a long time (with one of the
most seminal contributions being Ivan Illich in the mid-1970s,
of course (Illich, 1976), I think what you're saying in your previous answer is that although a Kuhnian 'scientific revolution'
is by no means imminent in the realm of modern medicine, we
do at least have quite an advanced understanding of why it is
that the current mainstream biomedical paradigm is grossly inadequate, and abysmally fails to describe and understand reality and *life itself* in a way that would render its medical 'treatments' appropriate and in tune with living realities, rather than
being routinely iatrogenic.

So, as you write, Thomas, we have to fundamentally re-think
our habitual *causal attributions* – for example, as you say,

The root cause is not the microbe as a point, but in the
periphery of the interrelationships that we ourselves have
caused. …[A]ll micro-organisms… are only to be understood as part of a larger whole, and therein will lie the
paradigm shift. To think in a living way means to think anew
every time, because the current contexts are always new.

As well as being a 'science of living connections' (your
beautifully evocative term), this also strongly suggests that a

71

'post-revolutionary' holistic medical science will also be one which has *uniqueness and individuality* as a core organising ontology, as opposed to the normalising monocultural bludgeon of Industrial-Complex biomedicine. And I also wonder whether our mainstream, 'normal-science' understanding of existing mechanistic conceptions of 'causality' itself, and of scientific 'explanation', will themselves also need to be fundamentally re-cast (which can only surely happen if the ideologies of patriarchy, determinism and the accompanying Victimhood Archetype are also problematised and transcended – themes we touched on earlier).

I'm also wondering whether a genuine 'scientific revolution' in medicine will necessarily require paradigmatic insights and breakthroughs that have literally never been thought before – or whether the seeds of the paradigmatic revolution that needs to happen might already be nascent in some of the ideas and insights of (to take just some examples) philosophers like A.N. Whitehead and Charles Hartshorne, process philosophy and the process theory of 'post-modern' medicine; Rudolf Steiner, anthroposophical medicine and Goethe's holistic scientific approach; great thinkers like Martin Heidegger, Georges Canguilhem, Hans-Georg Gadamer, Huston Smith, David Bohm and Rupert Sheldrake; philosophical vitalism and panpsychism; psychosomatic medicine and the 'mysterious leap from the mind to the body' of psychoanalysis (e.g. Deutsch, 1959; Erskine & Judd, 1994); and functional medicine, environmental medicine, person-centred medicine, and so on. Or in other words, to what extent are the seeds of what a new, viable medicine will look like *already available* and waiting to be assembled in this vast body of alternative ways of thinking about human health, illness and healing? Or will quite new epistemological and ontological breakthroughs and discoveries (also) be needed?

I'm also aware, finally, that 'revolutionary' changes in science and culture can't be understood or predicted without locating them in the wider *evolution of human consciousness* (Crook, 1980; Tarnas, 1991). These are big questions, I know! – but I also know that you'll have a lot to say about these momentous issues, Thomas.

TH: Basically, all the questions we are addressing here revolve around the age-old body–soul problem. Because we are not prepared to solve it, or because we have not managed to resolve the fatal Cartesian dualistic dilemma through the Enlightenment, that is why psychosocial catastrophes such as the Corona crisis are developing. We have created an abstract viral parallel world that is completely disconnected from human reality, and which is now taking on the life of a monster.

The earth and the human being are a common reality: 'the world is organised towards subjectivity' (H.-G. Gadamer, *mutatis mutandis*),[56] everything we separate out of the great context of this primordial symbiosis, everything we dis-integrate, becomes a source of error, even of a destructive nature.

Those who talk about viruses by invoking parasitic-enemy images make them the projection field of their own fears and their latent militaristic mental attitude, and in doing so overlook their deep co-evolutionary connection with the human being (right down to mental processes!); and moreover, they create a kind

56. Quotation adapted from Hans-Georg Gadamer (1900–2002), a highly influential German philosopher in the continental tradition, best known for his 1960 magnum opus on hermeneutics, *Truth and Method* (Wahrheit und Methode). His influential book on medicine, *The Enigma of Health: The Art of Healing in a Scientific Age*, was published by Polity Press (Cambridge) in 1996. On Gadamer and subjectivity, see Bernet, 2005. On Gadamer's view of medicine as a *dialogical* process, see Abettan, 2016.

of phantom, a spectre that menacingly haunts us.

I think the most important thing we have to achieve in natural science today is an integrative understanding of evolution. Paracelsus[57] already put it this way: 'Nature is made up of letters, and the word that designates them is man'. This fundamentally important idea can be traced today to all microbiological and genetic processes. One of the leading microbiome researchers in Germany, Thomas Bosch from Kiel, has illustrated this very clearly in his book *Der Mensch als Holobiont* (in translation, Man as a Holobiont). And the virologist Karin Mölling describes the human genome as a 'colourful potpourri from the gene pool of the entire earth'.

We share at least 80 per cent of our genetic material with horses – but that is only the external view of a phenomenon that also has its inside view: the common history of humans and horses, their deep soul relationship and their eco-cultural co-evolution. The horse is in us, not only genetically but in a soul-resonant relationship. The horse touches us because we carry 'equine' within us. Like is only recognised by like (Empedocles).[58] We would not be able to love these noble creatures if there were not a deep soul-like kinship with them by nature.

There is a fascinating new science called psychomicrobiology (see Anderson et al., 2017), which reveals connections previously thought to be unthinkable between gut bacteria and our mental states and cognitive abilities. As with horses, we share

---

57. Paracelsus (1493–1541) was a Swiss physician, alchemist, lay theologian and philosopher of the German Renaissance. See, for example, Di Stefano, 1994.
58. Empedocles (494–434 BC) was a Greek pre-Socratic philosopher, best known for originating the cosmogonic theory of the four classical elements. He also proposed forces he called Love and Strife, which would mix and separate the elements.

an ancient history of co-evolution with micro-organisms; we have gone through countless metamorphoses with them. We could continue the narrative of connections endlessly.

'The whole earth is human!' – this sentence is not an attempt to revive a romanticised nineteenth-century view of nature, but merely describes the logical inversion that humans are a compendium of all natural phenomena. We are interspersed with viral, bacterial, plant and animal genes; and what we have here before us as a biological fact, we need only translate into the language of the soul and spirit, for there, the same principles and forces are at work, only on different levels of description. Today we cannot yet clearly describe the 'anatomy' of the feeling for the horse, because our spiritual sensitivity is not yet sufficiently finely and consciously developed for this. But what Greek mythology experienced and described as the Centaur we will perhaps grasp anew in the future, with a finer depth of focus of the psychological-scientific gaze.

The physicist Hans Peter Dürr once summed up our central epistemological dilemma thus: 'We have completely disassembled the world and now we have the problem that we can no longer put it back together' (see Dürr, 2010).

I would like to briefly touch on a second point of our theme. What was described in myth in the ancient world of the Greeks as the Titan Chronos is currently experiencing the first birth pangs of a modern scientific renaissance: the rediscovery of time! Time precisely is *not* conceived as an abstract physical unit of measurement, but as the 'fabric' from which all living things are woven. Thus, every organism is permeated by structured time and all the regularities that are evident in chrono-biological orders (every animal and every plant is the result of a time choreography – the hoof of the horse corresponds to the nail of the human middle finger, but emerged from a different developmental dynamic) are also at work in the creative workshops of human 'world interiors' (Rilke).

In recent years, modern physics has declared time to be an illusion because it cannot be grasped on the physicalist level. We cannot even comprehend time as a physical quantity because it is a phenomenon of the living. The key to the body–soul problem lies in the essence of time, but only the experience of our own reflection can teach us about this phenomenon. The experience of the pure process, the pure activity within, in thinking, is the same as that which we find, for example, in a living cytoplasm.[59] In every cell, hundreds of thousands of metabolic processes take place simultaneously every second. When we write endless chemical formulae on the blackboard, it is only an attempt to present this purely processual phenomenon in such a way that we can better understand it with our naïve, building-block thinking.

It is some 300 years of materialistic thinking exercises that have deeply imprinted themselves in people's brains, so that today we can no longer think the purely living. In his work *Das Prinzip Leben* (The Principle of Life), which is well worth reading, Hans Jonas writes that the ancient Greeks could not actually think of death at all: their world was immersed in a single animated aliveness, and everything was filled with soulful beings and gods. Today it is the other way round: we have created a dead, mechanistic universe and no longer understand the living, with life itself having become the central enigma of all science.

On the scientific side, I see microbiome research as a light on the horizon. Because micro-organisms are very close to the

59. Cytoplasm is a jelly-like substance between the nucleus and the cell membrane.

purely processual understanding I mentioned earlier, they will force upon us a completely new dynamic of thinking; otherwise, we will no longer understand anything at all in this regard, for the traditional, analytical methodology completely fails here. I think that in the next few decades the paradigm shift *will* take place, and we will experience a new 'love affair' between natural science and the humanities. We will recognise that the same laws are inherent in our thinking as they are in living nature:

> ...nature, I was convinced, is made in such a way that it can be understood. Or perhaps I should more correctly say the other way round; our faculty of thought is made in such a way that it can understand nature.... It is the same ordering forces which have formed nature in all its forms and which are responsible for the structure of our soul, and therefore also of our faculty of thought. (Heisenberg, 1969, p. 123 f)

Forty-five years earlier Rudolf Steiner formulated it in a very similar way: 'It is of the greatest importance to know that the ordinary thinking forces of man are the refined forces of formation and growth' (Steiner & Wegman, 1991, p. 12). In this lies a core insight for overcoming dualism.

RH: There's much I'd like to pick up on from this wonderful answer, Thomas – for example, in relation to 'the body–soul problem', time, the nature of human thinking and our inability to 'think the living' (your evocative phrase), the ways in which our modernist materialist cosmology has de-animated the world into 'a dead, mechanistic universe', the paradigm-transforming potential of processual microbiome research, and so on. And with regard to what you term the 'purely processual phenomenon' that 'in every cell, hundreds of thousands of metabolic processes take place simultaneously every second': how on earth can reductionist science and simplistic causal thinking ever imagine that they can get *anywhere near* a remotely viable, realistic account of that reality with their blunt analytical instruments, without doing a kind of terminal violence to it? The term 'modernist scientific hubris' comes to mind.

But if I may, in my next question I'd like to return to the issue of *stress and fear* in relation to illness which we've briefly touched upon already – as it seems to be such an apposite litmus-test as to how and why allopathic biomedicine can be just plain wrong (or at best hopelessly partial to the point of caricature), *scientifically* speaking. I've recently been reading your enthralling 2020 article 'The corona syndrome: why fear is more dangerous than the virus' (Hardtmuth, 2020b). In that article, you refer to the 'chaos [that] is caused when fear, ignorance, panic and unscrupulous business interests coalesce and run out of control' (ibid., p. 13). There's enough material for a whole conference there alone!... And deepening your analysis of the fear question, and no doubt underpinned by a far more holistic understanding of how psychosomatic, 'body–soul' processes occur, you then write the following:

> ...viral activity increases in every ecological system… as soon as this system comes under stress…. If the organism becomes stressed…, the dormant state can become lytic (destructive), which means that the virus starts to multiply and destroy the cell (Lysis). We then have an infectious disease…. *The most significant cause of human illness is chronic, negative and fear-induced stress!....* When self-confidence is lost through fear and shock and with it the motivation to live, we withdraw from life as human beings *and our immune system collapses.* (ibid., pp. 17, 18, my italics)

You also quote G. Hüther thus: 'Fear… interferes with the regulatory system at the centre in the brain stem that integrates and guides bodily reactions and therefore the self-healing capacity of the organism'. And you quote a 2007 empirical study by

Cohen and others (presumably just one of many similar studies),[60] showing the impact on the immune system of being unemployed. These empirical findings are entirely consistent with the aggregative data estimating that the global mortality rate rose by hundreds of thousands in the 2010s due to neoliberal Western governments' economic austerity policies (see, for example, Vlachadis & others, 2014; Standring & Davies, 2020; and McGrath et al., 2016). Indeed, the recommendations of the McGrath et al. study included the following: 'It is crucial that policy makers consider the psychological impacts of current and future policies. Creating the conditions for well-being and resilience directly helps to reduce distress both in the short term and the long term' (ibid., p. 1). And with direct relevance to the imposed Covid-19 regulations to which the global population has been subject, McGrath et al.'s exhaustive literature review identified five specific ways in which austerity policies negatively impacted mental health: humiliation and shame; fear and mistrust; instability and insecurity; isolation and loneliness; and being trapped and powerless. From this, it appears that, psychologically speaking, it would have been difficult to design Covid-19 regulations that were more damaging than those that governments across the globe chose to impose in lockstep.

And so the corollary of all this: 'Societies... in which people are not anxious but courageous, creative, cooperative... do not provide a fertile soil for epidemics' (Hardtmuth, op. cit., p. 18). At this point, I can offer a personal experience of this phenomenon. I have been part of a substantial activist group that throughout the 'pandemic' has not observed the social-distancing and mask regulations, has had regular close contact, and which to a person has not been consumed by fear of 'the virus'. Now if the mainstream, simplistic germ-theory narra-

60. See, for example, Ross-Williams, 2020.

tive about Covid susceptibility peddled by the UK government and their scientific advisors were remotely true, we would have been dropping like flies; but in reality, as I write (late 2021) *not one of us has contacted Covid, or any other illness, for 18+ months*. And we are by no means all spring chickens, or lacking in potential co-morbidities! This anecdote seems to be entirely consistent with what you are saying here about fear and stress, and their self-fulfilling, illness-generating nature.

Now would I be somewhere near correct in saying that this is the clearest possible example of just how wrong the prescriptions based on biomedical science can be when that science adopts its narrowly conceived pathogen and germ theory ontology? So in the case of the Covid-19 so-called 'pandemic', for example, we were told that all the restrictions imposed (and the accompanying fear-inducing propaganda to which citizens were deliberately subjected by government and mainstream media – Dodsworth, 2021; Brinton, 2021) were designed to *protect* us from the virus and limit its spread. Whereas on your analysis, these so-called protective measures had *precisely the opposite effect* to that which government and their scientific advisors were claiming; i.e. the amount of fear (even *terror*) that was generated (which I have to say was enormous, and quite unprecedented in the UK in my lifetime) was *itself* a major cause of increasing people's susceptibility to contacting Covid, and thus in many cases dying as a result. **In other words, people were at least as much *killed by fear* as they were by Covid-19 per se – and quite possibly far more so**.

If this is anything like true scientifically speaking, then it surely constitutes a scientific, cultural and political scandal of unimaginable proportions – perhaps, even, a state- and corporate-engineered crime against humanity. It would be good to hear both your view on this specific issue, Thomas, but also what you see as the wider paradigmatic learning it might hold for currently prevailing mainstream approaches to modernist science, and its robotic, positivistic use and deployment by politicians and policy-makers. In passing, I think your 2020 quotation is especially apposite here – i.e. 'The negative long-term immunological effects of the current [Covid-19] measures… are beyond the scope of statistical assessment' (Hardtmuth, 2020b, p. 19).

TH: I am grateful to you for raising the issue of anxiety, stress and illness, Richard; it is centrally important. We have already mentioned the three levels of autonomy – autonomy on the cognitive level, resilience on the psychological level, and immune functions on the organic level. All three levels cannot be separated, and they interact to a high degree. Today, in mainstream thinking the disease process is reduced purely to the biological level or to viral exposure, and this creates room for fatal errors – indeed, it is a criminal omission! People who hold this position, which also supports the whole Corona narrative, obviously have no idea about the close correlations between immune functions and psychological stress that psychoneuroimmunological research has brought to light over the last two decades (Schubert & Amberger, 2016).

We now know how directly interdependent our immune functions are with our psychosocial condition. When people are exposed to frightening impressions of horror and violence in front of the television, the drop in immune parameters can be measured directly; and the opposite occurs with positive or cheerful content. A study in *The Lancet* has indeed shown an enormous increase in mortality rates (HIV, suicides, infant mortality, etc.) in Greece in the context of EU austerity measures (Kentikelenes et al., 2014). Indeed, epidemiologists Kate Pickett and

Richard Wilkinson from London have shown how much population health depends on social balance and equity in a country (Wilkinson & Pickett, 2016).

It can be summed up in one sentence: *the human being is healthy where it is humane.*

Millions of ruined livelihoods, mass unemployment and poverty, a massive increase in mental illness, violence, fear, exclusion, and much more. All this Corona collateral damage will result in a collective *depression* of immunity, with corresponding consequences. If our media return to their legitimate profession – namely, that of presenting proper and objective information for people – it will become clear that the global Corona measures and their social consequences will claim many times more lives than the virus itself. In light of this, I object to the sweeping statement that people 'will *die from a virus*', as this is actually counter to human dignity.

When you deal with patients every day for 35 years and look closely, you get a feeling for why people die: from tiredness of being alive and from exhaustion and weakness, from lack of motivation in their lives, from the feeling of no longer being needed, or from social isolation – from depression, fear, grief and deprivation of love. I could share countless examples of this with you (Hardtmuth, 2020a). Sometimes the reason is not immediately evident, and only reveals itself through very intimate observation. If the immune functions weaken for the reasons we have mentioned, then naturally a 'foreign life' in the form of viruses and bacteria emancipates itself more easily. Cancer, too, is basically a matter of 'foreign autonomy' in the organism. A person does not die from a viral pneumonia – these are usually relatively harmless; but when he or she dies, it is usually down to a bacterial super-infection whose development is not due to the original virus, but to a weakened immune system.

What loneliness does to people has been demonstrated by the psychiatrist Manfred Spitzer from Ulm in his book published in 2018 (Spitzer, 2018). The risk of death from loneliness is higher than from smoking, alcohol and obesity. Until a few years ago, such things were not studied at all, so knowledge about these relationships is not yet widespread.

Richard, I would also like to ask you a question. On 1 August 2021 I took part in a demonstration against the Corona measures in Berlin, and I have never seen so many peaceful and relaxed people, families with children, pensioners, artists, musicians, intellectuals and even clowns – nearly all from the middle-class echelons of society, it seemed. I couldn't find a single 'Nazi' or other so-called 'radical', as they're so often presented in our media! Talking to some of the participants, it was so pleasant for me to experience how many sympathetic, courageous and also educated people there are in our country – a modern, colourful society, as one would basically like to see. In fact, the demonstration on the 'Straße des 17. Juni' and in the government district had been banned, so that the estimated 200,000 people dispersed in numerous smaller marches throughout the centre of Berlin.

What was frightening was the massive extent of the brutality and show of force with which the police acted. Endless squadrons of emergency vehicles raced through the city with sirens blaring and blue lights flashing – actually, completely senseless – generating a catastrophic kind of mood for which there was no justification at all. Countless police squads in black uniforms, with helmets, visors, batons, tear gas, firearms, knee and elbow pads (as if they wanted to win a war) obviously had orders from 'above' to stop and disperse the demonstration marches by means of numerous road-blocks. Some of the violence used was so martial in nature that the UN Special Representative for Human Rights Violations has since intervened with an enquiry to the government.

At one point, we were directly confronted by a chain of police officers. On closer inspection, the pale faces of totally over-strained and completely insecure young people, including many young women in their early twenties, who were sweating with fear, were partially hidden in these threatening-looking suits of armour; how grotesque! An older woman next to me obviously also made a similar observation, stepping forward and shouting to them, 'Why don't you take off your helmets – we won't hurt you!'. After this 'disarming' sentence, there was a short silence; it was one of those small profound moments where it brought tears to some people's eyes because this simple sentence had such a strong impact.

And now my question to you as a psychologist is: Where does this aggression and simultaneous fear come from, which threatens to divide society more and more at the moment, and which has already destroyed so many relationships in private life? Why do we keep losing our humanity in this field of tension of fear and power, although nobody actually wants that? Does the stoked fear of the virus generate an age-old social-psychological reflex – namely, that of 'solidarity out of fear', in which anyone who refuses this solidarity becomes a hate object, a 'covidiot', because he endangers the 'vital' cohesion of the group? How can we overcome these deep rifts and these radicalisations? What attitude do we need in order to maintain dialogue without risking our authenticity, or even denying our convictions and pandering to the mainstream, as is unfortunately very common right now?

The Austrian psychologist Alexander Meschnig recently wrote in a brilliant essay, 'The corona vaccination as communion', about the 'redemption' vocabulary with which vaccination is touted today as the only 'promise of salvation' (Meschnig, 2021). In turn, the Corona-deniers are associated with God deniers; that is, the propaganda perfidiously operates in relation to traditional religious processes and discourses, which of course in turn has the effect of reanimating archaic forces.

In my entire working and personal environment, I do not know a single Corona victim, and I take note of such socio-psychological pathologies with concern, even with a certain fear.

RH: I'm deeply moved by your description of the Berlin freedom march, Thomas; and I'm also so grateful that you have highlighted the highly complex question of why it is that people die. In your few words on this, you have comprehensively laid bare the hopelessly simplistic positivism of the mainstream narrative constructed around people 'dying from Covid'. The mainstream media's and Zombie science's hopeless conflation of dying *with* and dying *from* Covid-19 is bad enough; but the simplistic view that we can unproblematically categorise vast numbers of people as having 'died *of* Covid' is not only insulting to people's intelligence, but it so easily becomes a mindless mantra that people robotically repeat, as if it is an incontrovertible medical-scientific truth. Anyone who understands the dangers of ascribing uni-causal explanations for death knows that it is hugely more complicated than the grossly caricatured mainstream narrative is proposing with their simplistic statistics-for-the-masses.

Alexander Meschnig certainly makes an interesting point about 'redemption' etc. discourses being invoked in the Covid-19 era, as this is entirely consistent with, and deducible from, the way in which '*the* science' seems to have become the New Religion in modern culture – a phenomenon pointed out many decades ago by people like philosopher of science Paul Feyerabend (e.g. 1978).

You ask where 'this aggression and simultaneous fear come from' around Covid, and 'how we can overcome these deep rifts and these radicalisations'. And further, 'What attitude do we need in order to maintain dialogue without risking our authenticity, or even denying our convictions and pandering to the mainstream…?'. I think you're absolutely right when you say that 'the stoked fear of the virus generate(s) an age-old social-psychological reflex – namely, that of "solidarity out of fear", in which anyone who refuses this solidarity becomes a hate object… because he endangers the "vital" cohesion of the group'. I'll return to this phenomenon below in discussing the recent work of psychoanalyst and clinical psychologist Professor Mattias Desmet. And I think we can also throw much light on the 'aggression/fear' question by returning to the Persecutor–Victim–Rescuer archetypal drama triangle of Humanistic Psychology (e.g. Hall, 1993).

I think the name-calling trope 'anti-vaxxer'[61] illustrates the argument well. Having been repeatedly subjected to this offensive term myself, and having thought deeply how (if at all) to respond to such cancel-culture name-calling, it seems clear that this offensive term is deeply connected to *hate and victimhood*, and to the *closing-down of thinking*. More specifically, in Kleinian psychoanalytic terms,[62] hate is a pervasive phenomenon to which we are all subject; and it's one that is ripe for psycholog-

---

61. The German term 'Impfgegner' (literally, 'vaccine opponent') does not fully express the pejorative connotation in the English word.

62. Melanie Klein (1882–1960) was an Austro-British psychoanalyst. She is considered one of the pioneers of the psychoanalysis for children.

ical projection on to a 'hate-object' whose identity can easily be manipulated into existence by manufactured mainstream (medical, media and political) discourses, especially when fear and death anxiety are skilfully deployed at the same time.

The powerful dynamics of *blaming* are also deeply implicated in the 'anti-vaxxer' trope. In terms of the archetypal Persecutor–Victim–Rescuer drama triangle,[63] the incessant mainstream propaganda narrative has cleverly created huge numbers of unwitting **Victims** of the 'deadly', '**Persecutory**' virus. And once Victims have been thus manufactured (cf. Dineen, 1999), they will likely rage at anyone who threatens the very raison d'être and scientific legitimacy of their potentially life-saving **Rescuer...** – the 'vaccine'! And when all this is experienced as *quite literally* a matter of life and death, the very first casualty will be *the capacity to think*. Anyone who's been subjected to anti-vaxxer 'othering' and demonisation will have observed how the use of the term seems to render its deployers incapable of thinking beyond the trope's confines – and therefore also incapable of even discussing its legitimacy and origins as a descriptor.

Going more deeply into 'the psychology of Covid' (if I can call it that) for a moment – here are two apposite and telling quotations to begin with. Psychologist Carl Jung once said, '**People will do anything, no matter how absurd, to avoid facing their own souls'.** Early last century, H.L. Mencken, an American journalist, essayist, satirist and cultural critic, wrote in his *In Defense of Women*: 'The whole aim of practical poli-

---

63. The drama triangle describes a basic pattern of relationships between at least two persons, who take on the three roles of victim, perpetrator or persecutor, and rescuer, which has long been handed down in many fairy tales and heroic sagas. The model of the drama triangle describes how these roles are interrelated and how they are often alternated. See the Wikipedia entry on the Karpman drama triangle at https://tinyurl.com/2j6ssvfp – accessed 2 June 2022.

tics is to keep the populace alarmed (and hence clamorous to be led to safety) by menacing it with an endless series of hobgoblins, all of them imaginary.'[64] Mencken could have written these century-old words to apply in every last detail to the current Covid-19 era!

Based on the reasoning in Dan Gardner's interesting book *The Science of Fear: How the Culture of Fear Manipulates Your Brain* (Gardner, 2009), we can justifiably ask, what if people are exposed to unremitting news coverage of a 'deadly virus' allegedly (they are repeatedly told) killing large numbers of citizens? – with it being reported on every news bulletin, and being talked about on every blog, social media site and in all our conversations with family, colleagues, friends etc.? The effect is that many if not most of us will end up believing that there is a considerable possibility that we ourselves are at substantial risk of dying from this 'deadly virus' – whether this is objectively or factually true or not; and all the logical, rational, evidential reasoning in the world won't change most people's views on this matter, once they've calcified this view at a primitive emotional level. (I return to this phenomenon again below.) At worst, we actually create fictions that serve to buttress our belief that we are smart, moral and right – which, with grotesque irony, easily becomes a belief that keeps us on a course that is dumb, immoral, and factually wrong!

Gardner would also argue that *being afraid* is an ingrained biological feature of humankind. But *staying* afraid, on the other hand, is something over which we *can* have some conscious control. For Gardner, then, if we consciously know how it is that we make attributional errors, how we can be fooled into fearing things that we don't actually need to fear, then we at

---

64. Quotation sourced from https://tinyurl.com/4mv5wmry (accessed 1 May 2022).

least have the opportunity to better understand our own reactions to events, and so make better, more reality-centred decisions.

Combining Gardner's work with that of social psychologists Carol Tavris and Elliot Aronson in their book *Mistakes Were Made (But Not by Me): Why We Justify Foolish Beliefs, Bad Decisions, and Hurtful Acts* (Tavris & Aronson, 2015), we often find that when we leap to an immediate viewpoint that is emotionally driven rather than based on rational analytical deliberation, we are not only often unaware of this process, but when we do eventually look back at our decision(s) using analytical deliberation, we often use the faculty of reason to self-justify the decision that we originally made – *no matter how wrong it might be in reality* on any dispassionate analysis.

Tavris and Aronson also consider phenomena like people who refuse to consider any evidence other than that which supports the conclusion they have already reached, and those who take it as a professional slight if they're challenged to support or (heaven forbid!) reconsider their favourite theory! In other words, the phenomena of cognitive dissonance and *self-justification* – being, it's argued, normal and *necessary* facets of the human 'mind-brain' – **mean that once our minds are made up on a given issue, for all of us it is exceedingly difficult to change them.** And it also appears that anyone who is in a position of power is even more vulnerable to making these kinds of 'errors'.

Counterintuitively, moreover, we find that in the case of consistently replicated eye-witness memory research, the *least* accurate case witnesses tend to have the *most* confidence in the accuracy of their recalled memories! What a theoretical can-of-worms we have, then, when we try to make sense of how it is that people can hold such disparate views about the 'pandemic' with comparable degrees of sincerity and assuredness that they are right.

What is potentially useful about this perspective is that it shows how good people can do bad things – without necessarily needing to invoke deliberately bad intentions, or any 'conspiracy' to commit harmful acts. Thus, for Tavris and Aronson, although many of us hold the view that some people are basically bad and do things just to be evil, in reality most people who 'do evil' *themselves* imagine that they are doing good. Perhaps we even like to believe that the people we consider to be evil themselves know deep down that they are indeed bad. However, a more psychoanalytically informed view would argue that perhaps all human beings do possess *the capacity to commit evil acts*, if not be 'possessed' by evil per se (the explanation of which would need a whole other conversation!).

Tavris and Aronson suggest a two-step way out of this problem. First, one needs to recognise what is happening; but this is difficult because of our innate defensiveness in protecting the integrity of the self from the pain of cognitive dissonance. Secondly, we need to choose to stop the escalation of our delusional self-reinforcing narratives; but this is even more difficult, as it involves taking full 'adult' responsibility for what we have done, and facing up to the fact that we might not be the morally superior protagonist in the self-justifying story we've created. So it is perhaps far easier to articulate what needs to happen to get beyond our self-justifying polarised positions, than it is to specify how, precisely, such a shift can actually happen. Sobering indeed.

Perhaps even more pertinent to the discussion of fear and its effects is the recent work of psychologist Dr Mattias Desmet, a professor of Clinical Psychology at Ghent University, Belgium, who has conducted some very illuminating interviews on the mass hysteria that has been generated in the course of the Covid 'pandemic'. Desmet lectures in psycho-analytic psychotherapy and on the psychology of the crowd, with a master's degree and Ph.D. in clinical psychology, and a master's degree in statistics. His notion of 'Mass Formation' (a kind of *mass hypnosis*) is extremely instructive in relation to how the extraordinary extent of irrational, emotionally driven compliance that typifies the Covid-19 era was achieved.

Mass Formation (also termed 'crowd formation') is a specific type of group formation or 'group-think' emerging under very specific circumstances, with four pre-conditions needing to be met (Desmet with Lee, 2021; see also Desmet, 2022).

1. The lack of a social bond, or meaningful relationships in people's lives;
2. A pervasive lack of meaning in the world;
3. Free-floating anxiety in society which is sometimes difficult to explain; and
4. The presence of free-floating frustration and aggression.

Governmental and institutional responses to Covid-19 did indeed deliberately stoke primitive emotions (fear, hate etc.), with rational thinking being disastrously sidelined in the process. Throughout 2020–1, most policies and restrictions were based on fear and emotion, rather than on genuine scientific and/or medical reasoning – with 'The Science' itself being a major casualty of this process. Unethical professional psychologists working for governments deployed deliberate, well-documented techniques that artificially elevated levels of fear, and stoked shame and guilt – leaving many people in a state akin to hypnosis, unable to distinguish between propaganda and the real story and risks of Covid-19.

The aforementioned preconditions are sufficient for Mass Formation to take hold, then, once a suitable event triggers it. The catalyst in the Corona crisis was the manner in which Covid-19 was reported by government and a compliant mainstream media, with reporting deliberately utilising psychological techniques designed to change people's beliefs and behaviour without them being aware of it. Right across the globe, the mainstream media relentlessly pushed a narrative that repeatedly highlighted both an 'object of anxiety' ('the deadly virus', and a strategy for 'beating' it and 'making us safe'. In the Covid-19 Mass Formation, the media's manipulative techniques have included:

- **Disproportionality** – Relentless reporting on running death-count while ignoring protective factors like age, natural immunity and effective early treatments
- **Fear** – SAGE's Government advisors advocated hard-hitting emotional messaging to change the behaviours of those at minimal risk
- **Shame** – Ruthless shaming was deployed against anyone using their own judgement to protect their health
- **Guilt** – Children were deliberately targeted with a disgraceful 'killing granny' narrative

Whole populations were divided and terrorised by these media tactics – with the media also silencing and 'cancelling' any countervailing narratives – however distinguished and qualified the purveyors of such questioning narratives. The most terrified citizens then looked to media and government for comforting reassurance, demonising anyone questioning the official narrative. These schisms then generated a 'group-think' emotional environment, where terror based on exploiting people's death anxiety replaced rational thought.

Solidarity also played a key role in all this. With disconnected people suffering from free-floating anxiety all associating their anxiety with a specific object, a new *solidarity* emerged, where everyone buying into the narrative could identify and bond as part of this new social group. Even faulty strategies for dealing with the anxiety-object, championed by the mainstream media narrative, were willingly embraced to engender a reassuring 'solidarity' feeling that we are all dealing with the anxiety-object together. And

> regardless of how damaging the strategy may be, *people engaged in this new solidarity will feel better about their own anxiety* by simply engaging in a strategy (Mass Formation), regardless of the serious side-effects of such a poorly devised strategy that the mainstream media has created a narrative for. (Desmet with Lee, 2021, my italics)

And woe betide anyone who doesn't join in with the Mass Formation! – for 'if you don't, you are not showing solidarity to the new group that has been formed' (ibid.). It might even be claimed that all the measures allegedly designed to 'defeat' the anxiety-object 'are really just to prove to everyone else that you are a part of the new cult-like social group' (ibid.; mask-wearing might be a very germane example of this) At worst, all such measures 'succeed' in doing is identifying who is a part of their new cult-like social group, and little if anything more.

And finally,

> Because these people are hypnotised by the religious cult that they are now engaging in, any new science that conflicts with their current religious cult beliefs cannot be accepted. *They are closed off to new information,* no matter how definitive they [sic] may be. (ibid., my italics)

I think Professor Desmet's psychoanalytically informed Mass

Formation model throws much light on the psychological dynamics underpinning global Covid-19 hysteria. One thing seems clear. If we don't learn from this toxic history and become aware of the deliberate orchestration of Mass Formation to which whole populations across the globe have been subjected, we will almost inevitably repeat it in the future.

The *historical-cultural context* in which what I am calling 'Covid-hysteria' has unfolded is also relevant. Some 15 years before the Covid-19 era, a sociologist specialising in fear, Frank Furedi (2006), coined the term 'culture of fear', referring to 'the inflation of danger [in which] society today seems preoccupied with the dangers that people face. The past decade has seen a veritable explosion of new dangers'... – with the latter 'pal[ing] into insignificance in relation to the big threats, which are said to put humanity's survival into question' (Furedi, 2006, p. 28; see also Furedi, 2018). Furedi goes on:

> Our imagination continually works towards the worst possible interpretation of events. Expectations of some far-reaching catastrophe are regularly rehearsed in relation to a variety of risks... [including] – fears about an explosive epidemic of a lethal infectious disease..., with the inflation of danger now systematically pursued and widely believed. (ibid., pp. 28–9; again, note that this was written some 15 years ago as I write)

Furedi goes on to speak of a cultural consensus that

> humanity is in grave danger from a range of natural, social and technological factors, [with a] new genre of medical doomsday scenarios [giving] coherence to a new strain of panics about plagues and epidemics, which is spreading like wildfire through the worlds of science and popular culture.... Since AIDS..., there has been a series of dramatic encounters with infectious disease.... The most common feature of these disease scares is *the systematic exaggeration of the*

scale of the threat. (pp. 29, 30, my italics)

At the height of the 2003 SARS panic, for example, even when this 'terrifying disease' quite quickly fizzled out with just a few hundred deaths worldwide, 'alarmist accounts... continued to be circulated warning the public that SARS was the prelude to wave [sic] of new viral pandemics' (p. 30). One could perhaps be forgiven for the cynical conclusion that after so many false alarms and scares that fizzled out into nothing, the medical-industrial establishment were determined to ensure that Covid-19 was not going to join that disreputable list.

Furedi also cites Arno Karlen's book *Plague's Progress: A Social History of Man and Disease,* in which Karlen projected 'a massive global die-off' which, according to Furedi, 'might result from a "revived bubonic/pneumonic plague, a virulent new flu virus, a new airborne haemorrhage fever, or germs that lurk undiscovered in other species"' (quoting Karlen, 1995, p. 276). In *Plague's Progress*, Karlen interestingly shows that disease is a natural and necessary part of life; and how, crucially, whenever people make radical changes in their lifestyle and environment, disease tends to flourish – the implication being that we need to take greater care of our environment (as Terrain Theory would also strongly argue; see our earlier discussion).

I know that some commentators are making some tentative connections between the global roll-out of 5G technology and the incidence of Covid-19 (e.g. AZB, 2021; Warden, 2021, Fioranelli et al., 2020). I assume that the introduction of 5G technology (see Bevington & House, 2019–20) would constitute a 'radical change in environment', and that true scientists must stay open minded about any such possible relationships and do the requisite research, rather than deploying the 'conspiracy theory' trope with a knee-jerk rejection, and the resulting unscientific silencing, of any genuinely scientific investigation.

Resonating with the above discussion, Furedi is also withering about the media's deliberate manufacturing of fear (cf. Dodsworth, 2021 in relation to Covid-19). Thus he writes,

> the promotion of fear and propagandist manipulation of information is often justified on the grounds that it is a small price to pay to get a good message across to the public.... [So] rather than provide people with the information to make an informed choice, *everyone* is warned that they are at risk. (p. 33, my italics)

And more recently (Furedi, 2018, p. 102), he writes that 'there has never been so much propaganda warning the public about yet another danger to its health'. And it comes as no surprise that (Furedi again) 'scaremongering works most effectively when it enjoys the authority of science.... Fear appeals work best when they are able to draw on both the authority of science and the language of good and evil' (ibid., p. 134).

Some eminent journalists even support 'good lies' being propagated by the media that are allegedly 'for our own good': for example, with regard to AIDS awareness campaigns, eminent *Guardian* journalist Mark Lawson wrote in 1996 that 'the Government has lied, *and I am glad*' (pp. 33–4, my italics) – promoting 'exaggerations and inaccuracies' about AIDS. I hope readers will appreciate the great dangers of this slippery slope – especially in the context of an hubristic biomedical science that has total conviction in its own rightness.

On Furedi's view, then, it seems that Covid-hysteria was *an all-consuming epidemic of fear* that was just waiting to happen, the cultural preconditions for which existed – indeed, had been deliberately seeded – for many years before the advent of

Covid-19 itself, and for which one could even plausibly argue that humanity had been primed. To invoke a psychoanalytic term (that Furedi might well not approve of), Covid-19 could be characterised, at least in part, as an unconscious *acting-out of pre-existing* and carefully prepared existential angst, which was just waiting for an appropriate external 'object' on which to be projected.

So here we have a rich menu of psychological insights within a very specific psycho-cultural context, Thomas, that I hope throw at least some light on the question you posed to me! Please excuse the length of this answer, but your question has enabled me to stake out some key theoretical perspectives and wider concerns. It would be fascinating to hear your thoughts on any or all of the above, and the extent to which these insights and speculations resonate and dovetail with your own experience as a medical doctor, and whether a more complete (if complex) explanatory picture might begin to emerge from the coalescing of these more psychology- and sociology-informed ideas with your own medical perspective. Never, surely, was there more of a need for a holistic *bio-psycho-social-spiritual approach* to help us gain as full an understanding of the current conjuncture as possible.

TH: Richard, I am very grateful to you for your professional and very differentiated explanations, which are extremely helpful for my efforts to understand, because they put into a concise form what I have only vaguely seen myself. I am becoming more and more aware of how centrally important is knowledge of the bio-psycho-social effects of persistent anxiety in this day and age, especially for medicine.

In the context of my lectures, when it came to the topic of anxiety and its consequences for human health, I used to illustrate it to the students by way of an introduction with the following example. During the Korean War, 200 fallen US soldiers were once autopsied, all between the ages of 18 and 22, who had already spent several months at the war front with daily fear of death, and who then died in combat. In the autopsy findings, 77.3 per cent (!) of these young men had externally visible calcifications of the coronary vessels, and 15 per cent had at least one higher-grade stenosis that narrowed the lumen by more than 50 per cent (Enos et al., 1953). From my many years of experience in vascular surgery, I know that calcifications in the vessels do not actually exist in this age group. Only massive psychological stress over months can explain such findings in young people.

In the research laboratories of our industrialised medicine, no one even thinks to ask about such correlations. The discussion about arteriosclerosis revolves around cholesterol, diabetes and high blood pressure, etc. – all aspects that promise lucrative sales markets for corresponding long-term medications, but which miss the essential problem. Arteriosclerosis (heart attacks, strokes and other circulatory disorders) is a central medical problem mainly in the industrialised countries, and is also the most frequent cause of death in those countries. We know from the Tsimane, an indigenous people in the lowland jungle of Bolivia with very pristine, natural living conditions, that they have the lowest rates of arteriosclerosis and thus the lowest mortality from cardiovascular diseases worldwide (Kaplan et al., 2017). Against the background of modern knowledge showing that chronic stress and fear are among the main factors in disease aetiology, an open discussion about how we want to live at all, and how we imagine a livable, humane and less stressful future in a globalised world, would be a far more sensible act of preventative medicine than constantly fuelling new virus-fear scenarios that benefit the pharmaceutical companies but not people's health.

You speak of the exclusion (othering) of so-called 'anti-vaxxers'. This seems to me to touch again on a central point of our dialogue. In the past, the death of a close relative was at the top of the list of psychological stressors. Today we know that social exclusion, the experience of being devalued, is the most traumatising experience for human beings. Humiliation, degradation, embarrassment and, above all, the fear of losing that all-important sense of belonging have, as mentioned, a direct negative effect on people's immune systems. A meta-analysis of 87 studies has shown that social integration and support reduce the risk of cancer by 25 per cent (Spitzer, 2018: p. 151ff). This has also been shown in numerous animal studies; mice with cancer in social isolation have significantly accelerated tumour growth (Madden et al., 2013).

What I mean by this is that the long-term consequences of the psychosocial tensions created by the Corona measures – ever new epidemics of fear, constant harassment, exclusion and defamation of opponents of vaccination, anti-solidarity trends in society, social isolation through quarantine orders, unemployment, threats to livelihoods, chronic conflicts and ruptures in long-standing relationships – and the associated immuno-depressions cannot yet be foreseen in terms of their pathogenic effects.

The final balance of all these supposed 'protective' measures will ultimately bring to light an opposite effect. I only fear that the political zeal with which a critical reappraisal takes place – if it takes place at all – will be limited. There will probably be no media hullabaloo comparable to the Corona alarmism. All these negative consequences will not be attributed to the political measures, but to the virus or the pandemic in the sense of this constant distortion of the facts, which we are already used to from the Corona dramaturgy. A truly appropriate, constructive discourse oriented towards human reality and not towards the virological imperative seems to me to be increasingly distant at the moment; indeed, we are dealing with an increasing brutalisation of the communication culture; 'strong men' who loudly and insensitively proclaim simple truths and present themselves as doers and 'saviours' in the crisis are booming again today, as I write. 'When the sun of culture is low, even dwarfs cast long shadows', the writer Karl Kraus is said to have once said. This Corona crisis has created an anti-social climate that provides an ideal breeding-ground for the Mass Formation you mentioned (according to Professor Matthias Desmet).

But let us return now to the fear issue, and its medical dimensions. I would like to use the example of a skin disease like neurodermatitis to illustrate what a systems-scientific, integral medicine actually means. Millions of micro-organisms live on every square centimetre of our skin – bacteria, viruses, archaea, fungi… – without which our skin would immediately become 'ill'. It is like a micro-ecosystem that is organised or regulated in a highly complex, dynamic way. In addition to the micro-organisms, many other factors are involved: heat regulation, fat content, pH, salts, immune factors, hormones, the neuro-endocrine system and much more. The most important thing to consider now is the highly individual structure of this skin environment. Every person has their own unique skin flora. This is already being used today for forensic purposes; a microbial imprint on a PC keyboard can even be used to identify the last user after 14 days, with the same reliability as fingerprints (Fierer et al., 2010).

We speak of the skin flora, i.e. we can certainly compare this micro-ecology of the skin with the external flora; just as every location in nature has its unique character and harbours an individual composition of plants and animals, so there is a very individual, characteristic atmosphere on the skin of humans. Sniffer dogs can sense this 'microbial aura' up to many kilometres away.

If we disturb this milieu – for example, if a surgeon destroys all micro-organisms and also the acid mantle of his hands by sterile hand disinfection – then it takes a maximum of one day for the resident flora to be rebuilt and the original milieu to be restored. This example can be used to develop a dynamic concept of health. Health is not *a state*, but an ongoing individual *process*. Our skin environment is not just there, but is continuously created by us against external resistance. There are countless factors (anti-microbial peptides, antibodies and other immune factors) that do not fight the microbial communities on our skin, but individualise them: this is central to understanding viruses and bacteria. The more individualised and diverse the microbiome on our external and internal body surfaces, the less susceptible we are to parasites and so-called pathogens. In a recently published study, microbiome analysis of over 9,000 people aged 18 to 101 years of age found that the healthiest men and women, and those with the highest life expectancy, were those whose gut flora had changed or individualised the most over the years (Wilmanski et al., 2021; see also Zittlau, 2021, p. 20).

The skin is not a hermetic boundary between inside and outside, but a highly sensitive interactive milieu in which the inside and the outside flow into each other. This is the principle of perception when soul and world merge, the only difference being that on the skin, this fusion is realised biologically-organically in the form of the individual microbiome: it is part of the environment and the organism *at the same time.*

And now on to the phenomenon of neurodermatitis. As with other chronic skin diseases, the microbiome of the skin is severely disturbed in neurodermatitis, the biodiversity of the micro-organisms is considerably reduced, and there is a tendency towards pathological bacterial monocultures (e.g. *Staphylococcus aureus*). This also makes the skin more permeable, and we become susceptible to 'foreign life'. We can also say that the protective, individual 'warmth' environment is lost. How does this happen?

I'll describe it in a slightly exaggerated way. If a child has the need for closeness, warmth, touch and 'cuddling', but instead is cleaned, anointed, powdered and put into beautiful little dresses with hair bows every day in an almost sterilised bathroom, then a dissonance between soul and environment takes place. There can be numerous underlying psychological problems: maternal narcissism and inherited and pathological attachment styles, but also exaggerated fears that make mothers constantly fear the worst, what we also call 'catastrophising'. You yourself mentioned the inflation of dangers, as also described by sociologist Frank Furedi, which is one of the reasons why phenomena such as neurodermatitis have been steadily increasing for years. When the parents' fear overpowers the natural emotional bond with their child and the child receives more hygiene, medication and medical supervision than attention, when it is overloaded with more worry about all kinds of dangers than with trust and love, then over time this leads to the dysregulation of the skin environment. With real affection, the milieu of the skin changes immediately: it becomes warmer, the vessels dilate, the fine structures in the metabolism, even the electrical resistance of the skin change and, over time, even a different smell develops, which is essentially produced by the micro-organisms! (Human sweat is in itself odourless.)

With distant cold, the vessels constrict, the skin becomes dry and vulnerable, with burning and itching. Modern psycho-neuroimmunology now shows how the complex network of psychological, neuro-endocrine and immunological processes works in a bidirectional way between body and soul. In atopic dermatitis, a whole cascade of psychogenically induced inflammatory processes takes place, whereby the release of so-called stress mediators (noradrenalin, histamine and many other neuropeptides) puts the skin into a kind of permanent state of alert (Peters, 2020, pp. 79-107). The individualisation of the skin environment therefore no longer takes place properly, and that which generates warmth, our 'I' in its organic effect, withdraws because the 'contact' with the world takes on a cold and painful connotation – indeed, the skin becomes vulnerable, a place of complaint.

Richard, let me conclude this section of our dialogue by touching on a spiritual question. This may be very unusual in a microbiological context, but I would like to stimulate a thought in the readers that opens up a much wider horizon than this currently prevailing, old and fearful enemy-image of viruses; perhaps a kind of 'virosophy', we might call it.

We now know that viruses are the oldest, the most common, the smallest and the most diverse physical structures that life on Earth has produced. And now these viruses consist mainly of hereditary material – RNA or DNA. Viruses are the original form of everything genetic on earth, with all genes formed from viruses. All genes are composed of the four building blocks –

the nucleotides Adenine, Guanine, Cytosine and Thymine – whereby in RNA the Thymine is replaced by Uracil. Three such nucleotides each code for an amino acid, of which there are theoretically 64 (4^3), but *de facto* only 20. U-A-C, for example, codes for the amino acid tyrosine. This genetic code applies to all life forms universally on earth from the beginning, like a kind of primordial language. All proteins are composed of amino acids, so here too it is the case that a certain building-block sequence produces a certain protein quality. Instead of a building-block sequence, we can also speak of a script composed of four letters, or of a musical notation. At the Massachusetts Institute of Technology (MIT) in the USA, there are molecular biologists who assign a tone to each amino acid and thus produce a kind of protein music; this is called the sonification of amino acid sequences (Buehler, 2020). The analogy of the hereditary substance with a (musical) score has already given rise to numerous philosophical considerations.

Now, viruses have an enormously high genetic plasticity, with their genes constantly changing depending on the environmental context. Viruses can do anything with their genes: cut, duplicate, reduce, copy, recombine, transfer, and so on. In the extreme case, this means that a small virus whose genome consists of only 50 nucleotides has potentially 10^{30} ways in which it combines these nucleotides. The number roughly corresponds to the number of stars in the cosmos. With 1,000 nucleotides, this theoretical possibility reaches infinity. A coronavirus has a relatively large genome, with 30,000 nucleotides. The interesting question now is how these sequences are composed. Is it the virus itself or is it the context, i.e. the host organism or ecosystem in which the virus resides? The Corona crisis is dominated by a purely virus-centric way of thinking.[65]

---

65. Addressed in detail in my book *Mikrobiom und Mensch* (Hardtmuth, 2021).

So what it is ultimately about is the unlimited plasticity and diversity of viral genomes, which are ultimately also related to all the unlimited biodiversity of living nature. Without viruses, there would have been no evolution at all (Ryan, 2010). And now think of this building-block sequence as a kind of text, and compare it with human language or music. The scope for linguistic or musical forms of expression is just as unlimited as is the play of genes within the world of viruses. The sentence 'In the beginning was the word' takes on a peculiar new validity against the background of the viral primordial world. We must bear in mind that evolution spent by far the greatest period of time (about three billion years) on the development of microbial life before the first multicellular, i.e. visible, life forms emerged (about 600 million years ago). For three billion years, so to speak, 'the spirit hovered over the waters', a time in which the boundless 'wisdom' of all the metabolic processes emerged that can be found preserved in our organism today. The extremely complex visual pigments, for example, the so-called rhodopsins, which enable us to see in colour, were produced in the primordial sea by micro-organisms in a rich variety – we know of 700 different rhodopsins produced by marine micro-organisms.

The creative potential of nature has thus developed from viruses through countless evolutionary stages, up to the creativity of man and his very own boundless form of expression in language and music – a weird alpha and omega in the history of life.

> The most important formation of the dance of substances according to the music of the world is the protein, the protoplasm, as it is the basis of all living formation.... The cell came into being relatively late, as the last of the formations. It has never been the case that organisms have formed themselves out of cells; but the cell has only formed itself out of the living. (Steiner, 2009)

In Rudolf Steiner's time we did not yet know anything about viruses and genes, but we could certainly use the term 'virus' instead of 'protein' in the above quotation.

It only remains for me to hope that this crisis will provide the occasion for us to sit down together and think about many things in a completely new, systematic and thorough way.

RH: There's so much I'd like to pick up on here, Thomas. But as we're in the later stages of this wonderful conversation, I'll try to keep my points succinct. You've helpfully reminded me of something that came up earlier – i.e. the *standardisation* that is implicit and uncritically assumed in the methods and praxis of scientific medicine – specifically, when you write of 'the highly individual structure of [the] skin environment. *Every person has their own unique skin flora.*' (my italics)

The branch of psychology with which I predominantly identify, Humanistic Psychology, makes a great deal of the phenomenon of *uniqueness* – and yet mainstream 'industrial' biomedicine (if I can use that term) seems to me to implicitly assume that human bodies are essentially machines that all broadly function in the same way – and so, it's assumed, universal, essentially identical treatment protocols can be applied to all people (bodies), with little if any attempt to consider how the diversity and uniqueness that you refer to in your fascinating skin example might be relevant to the kind of the treatment that the physician offers.

This leaves me wondering, first, whether a key cause of iatrogenic medicine (i.e. medical treatment that does harm to the patient – e.g. Griffin, 1988) might stem, at least in part, from this industrial model of bio-medicine that assumes uniformity rather than uniqueness? And might it also be that one reason why complementary and 'alternative' medical approaches often provide something that mainstream medicine doesn't provide is that alternative approaches *do* tend to assume uniqueness in both the presenting ailment and in the person suffering from the ailment, instead of assuming uniformity and standardisation? And finally – and I realise what a huge question this is! – is it possible to begin to imagine what needs to change in modern medicine – both its process and its content – in order to make a shift from a uniformity ontology to a uniqueness ontology? I suppose that it's much easier, in one sense, to work with an industrial model – such that once a diagnosis is reached, little if any further thought and judgement is needed by the physician, as the treatment protocol for the diagnosed condition is laid down in the medical guidelines, and the physician then robotically follows the protocol. Is it any wonder, I'm now thinking, that there are such huge numbers of 'iatrogenic' casualties from mainstream biomedicine? I'd be really interested in your thoughts on all this.

Relatedly, I just mentioned the issue of *diagnosis*. If the problem with diagnosis in psychiatry and psychology is anything to go by, as outlined by critical psychologists like Mary Boyle (e.g. Boyle, 2007), then perhaps the *very notion of* diagnosis, and what it consists in, might need fundamental re-thinking and re-specification in a new medical paradigm. To be brief, in psychology, Boyle maintains that: diagnostic systems lack any scientific basis; diagnosis distorts the research process in a number of ways; diagnostic models seriously restrict prevention; and diagnosis is also ethically problematic. Of course there exists a very powerful *emotional* commitment to diagnosis by both physician and patient – with the physician experiencing the quasi-certainty and the alleviation of anxiety-generating uncertainty that diagnosis confers; and in the case of the patient, as Boyle writes:

...people may be helped or comforted by a diagnosis; they may (rightly) believe that a diagnosis means that some aspect of their problem has been encountered before or (wrongly) believe it explains their distress, or predicts its outcome, or that it excludes something worse. (Boyle, 2007, p. 291)

She writes further that (and my apologies for the long quotations):

It is difficult to overstate the amount of effort and money expended in making the diagnostic system look credible through, for example, the strategic misuse of medical and scientific language, concepts and analogies; a focus on reliability at the expense of validity; the false presentation of diagnoses as atheoretical ('just descriptions')...; and the extensive misrepresentation and omission in secondary sources of research data which do not fit the model. *There is, too, an important and growing symbiosis between the devisers of diagnostic concepts and pharmaceutical companies* in that diagnoses seem more plausible if there appears to be a specific drug to treat 'a disorder', while drug marketing is strengthened if there appears to be a specific disorder the drug can target. Diagnostic credibility is also fostered by popular habits of thought such as reification and question begging. (ibid., my italics)

And with regard to the convenience that diagnosis enables, Boyle writes:

Diagnosis also serves important administrative, professional, psychological and social functions unlikely to be served by alternatives. These include providing an apparently simple system for record keeping, financial management or access to services; ... allowing 'normal' people to locate irrationality in others, in a society which reveres rationality; seeming to solve problems of blame and responsibility; and distracting attention from the harmful psychological consequences of social and political policies and structures. (ibid., p. 292)

Of course Boyle is talking about *psychiatric* diagnosis here, but I imagine there could well be at least some cross-overs between her arguments about the fallacies of diagnosis in clinical psychology and psychiatry, and the case of mainstream biomedical practice more generally – for it is *principles and processes of assessment and categorisation* which are at stake here. I realise this opens up a new 'front' in our conversation, Thomas, but I think the issue of diagnosis is taken for granted far too much in mainstream biomedicine, and is far more problematic, both philosophically and in terms of its multiple effects, than is commonly realised. I wonder whether you agree?

Finally, can we return to the issue of *anxiety* and its medical/somatic effects? – as an instance of a wider paradigmatic question about the nature of medicine as a praxis. You refer to 'how centrally important is knowledge of the bio-psycho-social effects of persistent anxiety in this day and age, especially for medicine' – and your example from the Korean War is certainly a very telling one. As you say, 'In the research laboratories of our industrialised medicine, no one even thinks to ask about such correlations'! And further, you say that 'the long-term consequences of the psychosocial tensions created by the Corona measures… cannot yet be foreseen in terms of their pathogenic effects'. A chilling situation indeed.

All this seems to me to lead directly to the issue of *holism in medicine* – and the necessity of considering the body, the mind *and* the emotions – indeed, the soul and the spiritual dimension – in any thorough and *genuinely* scientific assessment of people's well-being and dis(-)ease. In my own field of the psychological therapies, there is some very interesting literature on psychosomatic medicine, and what psychoanalyst Felix Deutsch (1959) referred to many years ago as 'the mysterious leap from the mind to the body' – or 'conversion', referred to earlier (see also Stein, 1985; Taylor, 1989; Erskine & Judd, 1994). This is a body of literature which would certainly be very critical of a narrow biomedical paradigm in medicine, as well as of the Cartesian dichotomy between mind and body. Yet it would also be very aware of the dangers of an unbalanced, unholistic 'psychologising', as well as of over-medicalisation. Dorothy Judd, one of the editors of *The Imaginative Body*, writes in that book of how the therapist has to struggle 'to understand in the patient the interplay of physiological reactions (such as nausea) to disease or medication, and psychological disturbance manifested somatically' (Sinason, 1995: 132). This for me resonates with your reference to 'a dynamic concept of health; [for] *health is not a state, but an ongoing individual process*' (my italics). And your following example illustrates this beautifully:

> When... the child receives more hygiene, medication and medical supervision than attention, when it is overloaded with more worry about all kinds of dangers than with trust and love, then over time this leads to dysregulation (of the skin environment).

So my question is: to what extent do you think physicians practising today do pursue such a holistic, processual approach to treatment and healing? And to the extent that this isn't happening, can you see any way in which we can get from the existing narrow bio-medical pharmaceutical paradigm, and to the kind of holistic, processual paradigm that we both strongly favour? Some simple questions for you!... ;-)

TH: Dear Richard, you have again raised many essentially important points. First of all, I would like to go into the biomechanical uniformity model of industrialised medicine and the concepts of diagnosis and health.

The word 'diagnosis' contains the term 'gnosis' in the sense of knowledge, so 'diagnosis' means that one can get through the 'surface' of the mere findings to an overall knowledge of the human being and his or her illness. Diagnosis is more than a finding, but today, for example, a positive PCR test is turned into a diagnosis of Covid-19, although the person can also be completely healthy.

The recognition of disease basically presupposes the recognition of health. However, the question 'What is healthy?' cannot be grasped without a concept of the individual, because health is not normative, but rather, has a highly individual quality. I would like to take a closer look at this important point. The philosopher Hans-Georg Gadamer, whom I hold in high esteem, writes in his book *The Enigma of Health* (p. 96; p. 126 in my German edition):

> ... Health is something which somehow escapes [the objectifying scientific method] in a unique way. Health is not something that is revealed through investigation but rather something that manifests itself precisely by virtue of escaping our attention. We are not permanently aware of health, we do not anxiously carry it with us as we do an illness.... It belongs to that miraculous capacity we have to forget ourselves.

And further (p. 108; p. 138 in my German edition): 'If health really cannot be measured, it is because it is a condition of inner accord, of harmony with oneself that cannot be overridden by other, external forms of control.'

We are now witnessing certain political and scientific elites (like the World Health Organisation (WHO) and the World Economic Forum) presuming to define 'the good' for society or health for all. But there is a danger in an objectifying concept of health, which the author of *Corpus delicti,*[66] Juli Zeh, calls the 'danger of forced happiness', in her fictional novel that foresaw the health dictatorship that has now come to pass in an almost prophetic way.

The common WHO definition of health ('a state of comprehensive physical, mental and social well-being and not merely the absence of disease or disability') has repeatedly met with criticism, for example from the medical sociologist Alf Trojan and the psychologist Heiner Legewie:

> However, in view of the anthropologically inescapable threat to human existence through ageing, separation, loss and death, the guiding principle of 'comprehensive well-being' must appear problematic. Behind this idea is a belief in progress that sees human suffering as defeatable, an ideology that is criticised under the headings of healthism and fitness society. Suffering and life crises are not only fundamentally unavoidable, they not only bring with them an increased susceptibility to physical and mental illness, but they also represent indispensable impulses for personal development and the maintenance of health. (Legewie & Trojan, nd)[67]

Why is there no objective definition of health? Not only the soul and mind, but also the human organism is much more individual than we believed until just a few years ago, with epigenetic research showing more and more clearly that our individual behaviour, feelings and thoughts are also imprinted on our genetic regulation in the long term. The analysis of individual brain cells reveals an overwhelming variety of different gene structures: 'The genetic changes in my brain are unique. They only occur in my brain, not in yours' (neuroscientist Fred Gage,

66. A fictional novel published in 2010 that foresaw in almost prophetic fashion the health care dictatorship as it has now come to pass. (Zeh, 2010).
67. See Technische Universität Berlin, 2020, p. 3. The script in this online document is a slightly abridged excerpt (Chapter 2 and parts of Chapter 1) from Trojan & Legewie, 2000.

Californian Salk Institute in an interview with Deutschlandfunk – see Lange, 2016).

It is the same with the immune system, which can be described as a kind of 'fluid brain' that learns and gains experience in an individual way throughout life. Through the reductionist antigen–antibody logic, we completely overlook the fact that our immune system as a whole, as an organ, is constantly confronted with huge microbial ensembles, for example with the microbial 'aura' of a person in the context of a close encounter. This is like our brain, which integrates the millions of singular pieces of information with which it is constantly flooded into whole images and experiences. Our immune systems are shaped by very individual experiences, and also by how much activity, i.e. alertness and interest, we put into these experiences and how engaged we are in processing them.

The presence of our conscious awareness in life experiences equally stimulates our immune activity. We have to process new experiences – for example, a deception or manipulation at the level of consciousness – in the same way as we have to learn how to deal with a new virus or with an RNA vaccine – which basically also represents an attempt to deceive the immune system. Such learning processes can vary greatly from person to person.

And now we also find that microbial colonisation and its functional interconnectedness with our organism are unique to each person. Numerous drugs, for example, are metabolised quite differently by individual microbiomes, which challenges the common concept of standard therapies.

We've already mentioned that the individualisation of our microbiome is the essential protective factor against infectious diseases. The study by Wilmanski et al. (2021), referred to earlier, has shown this. Individuality or authenticity is basically the source of health.

In this context, there is another highly revealing study. In his study on autonomy training, the medical sociologist Ronald Grossarth-Maticek describes the Heidelberg Intervention Study, in which many thousands of people were observed regarding their health over a period of 20 years. On a certain cutoff date, all medical data (risk factors, current state of health, objective health factors such as normal weight, non-smoking, sport, healthy diet, etc.), as well as the ability to self-regulate, were recorded by a test procedure, and the study was repeated 20 years later. Self-regulation is understood as the ability to arrange one's life in such a way that one feels authentic and comfortable.

As expected, after 20 years in the study the healthiest participants were those with good self-regulation and all objective health factors. The worst performers were those who had neither. However, it was remarkable that people who did not have a single general positive objective health factor – i.e. who were overweight, did little sport, ate poorly and had poor hereditary factors, etc., but who had good self-regulation in that they were able to lead their lives in such a way that they could cope well with stress and felt balanced and coherent – had the same outcome after 20 years as those who had all the positive factors but had poor self-regulation (Brand Eins, 2002; see also Grossarth-Maticek, 2013). The inner warmth of authenticity, this feeling of being in tune with oneself, thus seems to be a basic foundation for health.

There are people for whom health becomes an end in itself. They do not pursue prevention out of the joy of swimming, hiking, cycling, etc., but out of an often fear-driven, exaggerated demand for performance from oneself, for which they constantly strive. They are in a constant state of worry about a life they never lived. They do not see their health as something that comes from themselves and their self-responsibility, but as a norm set from outside to which they have to conform.

> I refuse to define what health that is desirable for others should contain. I refuse to define health as a goal that can be defined by a third person. (Valentine Borremans)[68]

The biomechanistic uniformity model of industrialised medicine increasingly operates outside of the reality of people's lives. Diseases and their course are much more individual than we think they are, but no statistics can capture that. We only look at the virus and no longer at the human being.

We are currently witnessing the 'return of collectivism' in a new guise, according to philosopher of science Michael Esfeld writing on a new totalitarianism (Esfeld, 2021; see also Lütge & Esfeld, 2021).[69] Humanity is being persuaded that everyone is threatened by the same disease, which is caused by a single virus and can therefore only be treated with a single therapy strategy! This is the complete counterpoint of an individual medicine that is appropriate for humankind. Humanity is seen as a 'herd' to be immunised, and its individuals as uniform biological objects whose immunological deficiencies could be collectively corrected by a new pharmaceutical product.

A few days ago as I write, I had a conversation with a colleague whom I hold in high esteem. She told me about an elderly, sin-

68.   Valentine Borremans was director of the Center for Intercultural Documentation in Cuernavaca, Mexico and a collaborator of Ivan Illich's. Quoted from Illich's 1976 book.
69.   See philosopher of science Michael Esfeld on a new totalitarianism in Corona times – Esfield, 2021.

gle man who had also gone through a serious biographical crisis with his Corona disease and whom she stood by for weeks. She visited him at home every day and had long conversations with him because she was convinced that he could not get well without a human being as a remedy – and he did get well, and his doctor was more than a service provider at that moment; she had become a companion on his journey.

From a financial viewpoint, such behaviour is highly ineffective for a doctor today. If you ask to what extent doctors today are guided by a holistic and not by economically driven therapeutic considerations, then I have to say that there do still exist doctors who are with their patients with empathy and unconditional commitment; but

> …if economic interests override the need of the person concerned to such an extent that the sick person is not seen as a call for help but as a threat to the balance sheet, then this leads to an alienation of the helping professions from their own identity, thus plunging them into a crisis of meaning in their actions. (Maio, date unknown)

The old illusion that success, public prestige and wealth alone promise happiness is only still widespread amongst those doctors who do not know these deep existential experiences in the encounter with their patients, and their spiritual nature.

At the end of our conversation, the colleague said that the most important thing in a human life is basically our relationships, and that the Corona crisis is actually a call to grasp this truth anew. I could only agree with her.

RH: Given that our conversation is already over 20,000 words long, Thomas, I think I'd better – with great reluctance – make this my final question to you. I was interested in what you said about the phenomenon of 'diagnosis'. From what you say, I take it that the problem doesn't reside with diagnosis as a practice *per se*, but rather, with the narrow positivistic way in which it is commonly deployed in mainstream biomedicine – i.e. as a labelling exercise that, once the label has been applied, closes down rather than opens up deeper reflection on a given patient's illness and dis-ease. If it doesn't exist already, it would be good to see an authoritative 'new-paradigm' text that reclaims the notion of diagnosis from biomedicine's narrow colonisation and use of the term.

What a delight to discover that the great Gadamer is a favourite writer of yours! I have his book *The Enigma of Health* (from which you quote), and this got me wondering about medical training, and the extent to which trainings pay any attention to the deep philosophical and existential questions about which Gadamer poses such searching and intelligent questions. I sincerely hope a new paradigm for medicine would explicitly incorporate a consideration of such questions in its trainings, along with close attention being paid to psychosomatic medicine and the accompanying psychodynamics (Stein, 1985), the psychological complexities of doctor–patient relationships, and the place of spiritual healing in 'medical treatment'. But I wonder whether such shifts are remotely possible under the current biomedical regime? – and how this might change.

You refer to 'certain political and scientific elites presuming to define "the good" for society or health for all'; and you go on to refer to the danger of objectifying the concept of health, and Juli Zeh's notion of the 'danger of forced happiness'. I think this is a key issue that anyone concerned with human well-being needs to cast a critical eye upon. In the UK, the inexorable march of Cognitive Behaviour Therapy (CBT) as a modality of psychological 'treatment' (e.g. House & Loewenthal, 2008a, b) and the associated 'psychology of happiness' (Layard, 2011; Layard & Ward, 2020) constitute a clear case of what you're referring to, Thomas, with CBT being a classic example of the 'objectification of health'. On this view, then, well-being becomes *a technology* – and the French philosopher Michel Foucault has also written with great insight about what he terms modern 'technologies of the self' (e.g. Martin et al., 1998). I'm wondering to what extent there is any widespread knowledge and understanding within the medical world of these pernicious trends, and whether any critical literature exists on these questions that you might be aware of? If not, there surely needs to be!

What you say about numerous drugs being metabolised quite differently by individual microbiomes, individuality being the source of health, and diseases and their course being much more individual than we think they are – all this confirms my hunch that any true 'science' of medicine must embrace uniqueness as a core principle, rather than just assuming that standardisation is appropriate in medical treatment. Can you say something brief about what a new medical praxis that works in this way might look like? – a massive question, I know!

Finally, Thomas, is there anything you'd like to say to round off our conversation about the future of medicine, and your vision for how we might evolve from the overweening and hubristic pharmaceutical dominance of medicine to a medical praxis that is far more thoughtfully holistic in orientation?

Thank you so much for creating the opportunity for this enthralling dialogue, Thomas! I've learnt so much from your wisdom, and I know that anyone who takes the time to read this text will have a similar experience. My heart-felt thanks to you.

TH: Richard, before we conclude with your question of what a future individualised medicine could look like, let me first emphasise this important aspect regarding economics. The most important thing that the Corona crisis teaches us for immediate practice is that we need a complete decoupling of medical thinking from economic logic! Medical research must also be able to work completely independently of economic interests, otherwise this will lead to a creeping degradation of medicine.

The question of whether a person falls ill with an infection depends primarily on individual factors: constitution, disposition, self-regulation, psychosocial environment. Exposure, i.e. pure viral contact, plays only a subordinate role in the development and course of a disease; we are confronted with thousands of so-called pathogens every day; whether we become ill has very little to do with it.

Today's medicine, however, is making a gigantic worldwide effort exclusively in relation to exposure – i.e. masks, distance, hygiene rules, lockdowns, vaccinations, antivirals, etc. The decisive influence of individual factors is not even addressed in the public debate, let alone implemented in daily practice. Why is this so? Because our health systems are increasingly under the influence of economic strategies, and only those medical measures are favoured that keep this world's largest market – the health industry – running. No profits can be made with prevention, information, health education, stress reduction and the creation of humane, socially balanced lifestyles, but these would be the far more sustainable, salutogenetic measures in the long term. If the many trillions of euros that the crisis has cost so far had gone into ecological and social, i.e. people-oriented projects, it would have been a blessing for the whole earth.

Now to your question on what the future of a people-oriented, individualised medicine might look like.

I think all the questions and topics that we have dealt with so far in our dialogue, which has been so interesting and invigorating for me, ultimately revolve around one central question: What is a human being? A future medicine that is truly fit for human beings must ask itself this question again and again in all seriousness. It is true that we currently have a trend towards so-called 'personalised medicine', but this is oriented less towards the phenomenon of the uniqueness of each human being, and merely towards individually different biomarkers. Despite the personalised claim, this medicine remains trapped in the pharmaceutical logic of repair (Vollmann, 2013).

Perhaps the question of the nature of the individual can be clarified with the use of a metaphor. If one asks how many centres the infinite space of the cosmos has, then from a purely mathematically logical, external perspective, one must say: infinitely many! In reality, however, there are only as many as there are human beings. Every human soul is a centre of the world, a microcosm! But I don't mean this in the sense of a beautiful, philosophical Sunday speech, but as a concrete scientific task.

Earlier I mentioned Thomas Bosch, who describes the human being on the purely biological level of description as a *holobiont*, as an *integral of nature*. Rudolf Steiner calls the human 'I' the contracted cosmos. In concrete terms, this can be thought of as a process of inversion – i.e. just as in the inversion of a sphere the infinite periphery becomes the central focus, so in the human being the universal creative potentiality is germinatively predisposed (see Anon, 2022). Evolution works in an integrative way, i.e. what has gone before is always summarised in the new. Nothing is lost in nature; it only appears again and again in new forms.

The original biosphere of the earth lives on in us as a microbiome. Every human being carries, so to speak, the entire natural and cultural history as a predisposition or potential within him or her. All specialised abilities in the animal world are inherent as potential abilities in the human being – and this is also true for the spiritual potentials; one might say that the whole of heaven slumbers within us.

We all have a universal potential for development. Only when we work our way concretely into the phenomenon of the human being from this evolutionary-biological or evolutionary-psychological perspective can we develop any substantial concept of the 'I' at all. The creative universe scatters its own seed on the earth – that is the idea of the human being. In contrast, the idea of the 'I' as a neurobiological construct, as a self-model generated by the brain (Metzinger, 2009), which is widespread today, sounds like a kind of requiem for the human mind, which *abuses its freedom to explain itself away* (Safranski, 2016).[70]

The human being as a microcosm is basically ancient knowledge that we have to update today, right down to the scientific details. Medical students today are learning to think more and more from the whole to the part, but no longer backwards! The physicist Hans Peter Dürr, who has already been quoted in our dialogue, once said: 'Whoever insists on exactness must isolate and thus loses the context from which relevance can be inferred.' This sentence sums up our current situation: we analyse millions of molecules, viruses, genes and other biomarkers, produce a vast amount of data, numbers, statistics and test results; yet we have completely lost sight of the real existence of human beings oriented towards meaning and significance.

Medical education today needs subjects like philosophy of

70. Quoted in Scheurle, 2016.

science, epistemology, philosophical anthropology and hermeneutics as a basic psychotherapeutic principle – absolutely! Students today are virtually trained in the uncritical repetition of systems knowledge. Their own creative thinking is rather disturbing, but it is essential for the individual therapeutic process. We are currently experiencing the effects of years of such university 'conformity exercises', very clearly visible in these Corona times in the form of an almost soporific stereotype of the mainstream narrative.

Without a philosophical spiritual orientation, then, the ideal of the healing professions withers away, with which most young people originally started out, but of which there is usually not much left after a few years in the profession.

'What is an individual?', the evolutionary biologist Wolfgang Schad once asked. The truly perfect is the imperfect! The highest thing that nature has created is a self-creating, error-prone but *free* being. Therein lies what is human, that we stay in a common space of possibility, that we risk ourselves in the indeterminate or, as the sociologist Hartmut Rosa (Rosa, 2020) called it, that we live with 'unavailability', that we actively venture creatively into the open, as now in our conversation, but where we never know where it will go. The human ego is the current developmental event on this earth: each individual is a kind of bud on the family tree of evolution.

A person very close to me, with whom I could talk about everything, died a few years ago. When I was still a young student, we once sat together for a whole week at a quarry pond on our camping chairs and talked mainly about philosophical questions, every day until deep into the night, and there was not a single boring moment. This created an atmosphere that made me, as a young person, feel the infinite horizon of human – or, should we say, *interpersonal* – spaces of reality. For me, this was a very important, indeed a central, experience, and also for my later profession. Until two days before his death, I was able to talk to this person in this completely free way. It was always so interesting and invigorating that all fears of pain, suffering and death disappeared because they were simply not up for discussion. The psychiatrist Wolfgang Rißmann, following the philosopher Kierkegaard, called fear a vacuum phenomenon (see Rißmann & Pflug, (nd), excerpted from Adams et al., 2015), which only appears where the ego is not. This is a fundamental salutogenetic insight.

The ideal of a future medicine is 'talking medicine'. Getting back into conversation is basically the healthiest thing for human beings, and an elementary prerequisite for all healing.

Being me or being healthy is a lifelong activity against innumerable inner and outer resistances. Our biological self, the immune system, consists of many billions of immune cells and their cytokines (messenger substances), which have a half-life of only a few minutes, which means that we are constantly *re-creating* this biological self! And this also applies in a certain sense to our mental and spiritual activities, in whose environment the immune cells resonate as in a resonance chamber. The same individual force lives in our immune system that also inspires and shapes our thoughts and ideas anew every day.

We have talked about determinism, which makes human beings the victims of the most diverse powers: virological, biomechanical, neurobiological, genetic, depth-psychological, social, Darwinian, even spiritual determinism – we create them all ourselves in our thinking! We delegate power over ourselves to foreign entities, and thus carry forward old rituals of subjugation. Of course, we are determined to *some* extent by these things working from the past, but what is actually human works from the future as a vision, ideal or utopia.

When a person is depressed, we usually look for the causes in the past – which of course has its justification; we ask where from, but not where *to*. Depression tells me that something is wrong. Something is working in me from the future, the depression is the expression that this new other that is working is not yet there. We have to take this perspective in *all* therapeutic procedures – i.e. where does this person want to go? A very helpful question to ask a patient is always: 'What do you personally think would be the best way for your recovery?' With this question, the therapeutic dialogue can be opened, which is now less attached to the cancer cell, the virus or any 'diagnosis', but is primarily oriented towards the 'I' of the person and his or her reality of life. The Scottish psychiatrist Ronald D. Laing made this immediacy and presuppositionlessness of interpersonal experience the foundation of every therapeutic process – the human being as a remedy! Essentially, this latter should be the guiding star of medical thinking.

Richard, let me conclude by mentioning again another aspect in response to your question of what a new medical practice that works in this way might look like. The most important thing that the Corona crisis teaches us: *we need a radical decoupling of medical thinking from economic logic!*

I wish to repeat this because it is so important. The question of whether a person falls ill with an infection depends primarily on individual factors: constitution, disposition, self-regulation, psychosocial environment. Exposure, i.e. pure viral contact, plays only a subordinate role in the development and course of a disease; we are confronted with thousands of so-called pathogens every day, and whether we become ill has very little to do with it. And if the many trillions of euros that the Corona crisis has cost so far had gone into ecological and social – i.e. human-oriented – projects, it would have been a blessing for the whole earth.

Dear Richard, I would like to thank you very much for this conversation, and wish you all the best for the future.

Bibliography

Abettan, C. (2016). Between hype and hope: what is really at stake with personalized medicine? *Medicine, Health Care and Philosophy,* 19: 423–30.

Adams, K, Rißmann, W. & Roknic, M. (2016). *Das innere Gleichgewicht finden, Seelenübungen für Achtsamkeit, Herzenskultur und Willensstärkung* [Finding Inner Balance, Soul Exercises for Mindfulness, Heart Culture and Strengthening of Will]. Berlin: Verlag Gesundheit Aktiv.

Anderson, S.C., Cryan, J.F. & Dinan T. (2017). *The Psychobiotic Revolution: Mood, Food, and the New Science of the Gut–Brain Connection.* Washington, D.C.: National Geographic.

Anon (2022). Sektion für Landwirtschaft: Stream 6 Aesthetics and health – curative energies from the microbiome (EN). 4 February; available at https://tinyurl.com/2p835eky (accessed 5 May 2022).

AZB [Anon] (2021). Covid is the body's response to toxic poisoning. Independent Viewpoints website (independentviewpoints.net); available at https://tinyurl.com/3p9s3tyw (accessed 10 October 2021).

Bernet, R. (2005). Gadamer on the subject's participation in the game of truth. *Review of Metaphysics,* 58 (4): 785–814.

Bevington, M. & House, R. (2019–20). 5G technology demands a precautionary approach: an interview with Michael Bevington. *AHPb Magazine for Self & Society,* 4; available at https://tinyurl. com/4he84944 (accessed 1 May 2022).

Bosch, T.C.G. (2017). *Der Mensch als Holobiont. Mikroben als Schlüssel zu einem Verständnis von Leben und Gesundheit* [The Human Being as a Holobiont: Microbes as the Key to an Understanding of Life and Health]. Kiel: Verlag Ludwig.

Bosch, T.C.G. (2020). Die mikrobielle Vielfalt erhalten. Hygienemaßnahmen im Rahmen der Covid-19 Pandemie [Preserving microbial diversity. Hygiene measures in the context of the Covid 19 pandemic]. *Pharmazeutische Zeitung Prisma,* 27: 207–10.

Boyle, M. (2007) The problem with diagnosis. *The Psychologist,* 20 (5): 290–2.

Brand Eins (2002). Wo das Dogma beginnt, ist das Leben am Ende [Where

dogma begins, life ends]. Archived, available at https://tinyurl.
com/5d2ct6ru (accessed 2 July 2022).

Brinton, R. (2021) Book review essay of Dodsworth, 2021. *New View*
magazine, 100 (Summer): 88–93.

Brown, M.J. (2021). Against expertise: a lesson from Feyerabend's
Science in a Free Society? In K. Bschir & J. Shaw (eds), *Interpreting
Feyerabend: Critical Essays* (pp. 191–212). Cambridge: Cambridge
University Press.

Buehler. M.J. (2020). Sonification of the coronavirus spike protein (Amino
Acid Scale). Available at https://tinyurl.com/28nw5fsv (accessed 5
May 2022).

Černič, M. (2018). *Ideological Constructs of Vaccination*. Newcastle Upon
Tyne: Vega Press.

Clemens, V., Huber-Lang, M., Plener, P.L. & others (2018). Association of
child maltreatment subtypes and long-term physical health in a German
representative sample. *European Journal of Psychotraumatology*, 9
(1): 1510278; available at https://tinyurl.com/22d73xmr (accessed 5
July 2022).

Cohen, F. & others (2007). Immune function declines with unemployment
and recovers after stressor termination. *Psychosomatic Medicine*, 69
(3): S 225–34.

Crook, J. (1980). *The Evolution of Human Consciousness*. Oxford: Oxford
University Press.

D'Arcy, P.F. & Griffin, J.P. (1979). *Iatrogenic Diseases*, 2nd edn. Oxford:
Oxford University Press.

Desmet, M, with Lee, D. (2021). Totalitarianism in the world – Professor
Mattias Desmet. Available at https://tinyurl.com/ykj8uyv5 (accessed
1 May 2022; full interview available at this link).

Desmet, M. (2022). *The Psychology of Totalitarianism*. White River
Junction and London: Chelsea Green Publishing.

Deutsch, F. (ed.) (1959). *On the Mysterious Leap from the Mind to the
Body: A Workshop Study on the Theory of Conversion*. New York:
International Universities Press.

Deutschlandfunk (2022). Genom in Aufruhr: Der Mensch ist genetisch
instabil [Genome in turmoil: humans are genetically unstable]. 8
March. Available at https://tinyurl.com/3ypy48b4 (accessed 5 May
2022).

Di Stefano, V. (1994). Paracelsus: Light of Europe – a brief history.
Australian Journal of Medical Herbalism, 6 (1): 5–8; 6 (2): 33–6; 6
(3): 89–92.

Dineen, T. (1999). *Manufacturing Victims: What the Psychology Industry Is*

Doing to People. London: Constable.

Dodsworth, L. (2021). *A State of Fear: How the UK Government Weaponised Fear during the Covid-19 Pandemic.* London: Pinter & Martin.

Dürr, H.P. (2010). *Geist, Kosmos und Physik: Gedankenüber die Einheit des Lebens* [Mind, Cosmos and Physics: Thoughts on the Unity of Life]. Amerang, Germany: Crotona Verlag GmbH.

Engel, G.L. (1977). The need for a new medical model: a challenge for biomedicine. *Science,* 196 (4286): 129–36.

Enos, W., Holmes, R.H. & Beyer, J. (1953). Coronary disease among United States soldiers killed in action in Korea: preliminary report. *Journal of the American Medical Association (JAMA),* 152: 1090–3.

Erskine, A. & Judd, D. (eds) (1994). *The Imaginative Body: Psychodynamic Therapy in Health Care.* London: Whurr.

Esfeld, M. (2021). Die Rückkehr des Kollektivismus [The return of collectivism]. 21 October; available at https://tinyurl.com/ft6uyy94 (accessed 5 May 2022).

Feyerabend, P. (1975). How to defend society against science. *Radical Philosophy,* 11: 3–8; reprinted in N. Warburton (ed.), *Philosophy: Basic Readings* (pp. 261–71). London: Routledge, 1999; available at https://tinyurl.com/4zv28m5c (accessed 27 June 2022).

Feyerabend, P. (1978). *Science in a Free Society.* London: Verso Books.

Feyerabend, P.K. (2001). *Conquest of Abundance: A Tale of Abstraction versus the Richness of Being.* Chicago: University of Chicago Press.

Feyerabend, P. (2011). *The Tyranny of Science.* Cambridge: Polity.

Fierer, N., Lauber, C.L., Zhou, N. & others (2010). Forensic identification using skin bacterial communities. *Proceedings of the National Academy of Sciences of the United States of America (PNAS),* 107 (14): S. 6477–81.

Fioranelli, M., Sepehri1, A., Roccia1, M.G., Jafferany, M., Olisova, O.Y., Lomonosov, K.M. & Lotti, T. (2020). 5G technology and induction of coronavirus in skin cells. *Journal of Biological Regulators & Homeostatic Agents,* 34 (4); available at https://tinyurl.com/ynpkv5tx (accessed 10 October 2021)

Furedi, F. (2006). *Culture of Fear Revisited: Risk-taking and the Reality of Low Expectations,* 4th edn. London: Continuum.

Furedi, F. (2018). *How Fear Works: Culture of Fear in the 21st Century.* London: Bloomsbury Continuum.

Gadamer, H.-G. (1996). *The Enigma of Health.* Stanford, Calif.: Stanford University Press.

Gardner, D. (2009). *The Science of Fear: How the Culture of Fear*

Manipulates Your Brain. New York: Plume.

Gordon, T. (2015). Paul Feyerabend complains that science has authoritarian tendencies; is he right? Researchgate.net, July; DOI: 10.13140/RG.2.1.3358.5760. Available at https://tinyurl.com/ y5xdxyyk (accessed 20 October 2020).

Griffin, D.R. (1988). Of minds and molecules: postmodern medicine in a psychosomatic universe. In D.R. Griffin (ed.), *The Reenchantment of Science* (pp. 141–63). Albany: State University of New York Press.

Grossarth-Maticek, R. (2013). *Autonomietraining: Gesundheit Und Problemlösung Durch Anregung Der Selbstregulation* [Autonomy Training: Health and Problem Solving by Stimulating Self-regulation]. Berlin: de Gruyter.

Hall, J. (1993). *The Reluctant Adult: The Problem of Choice.* Bridport, Dorset: Prism Press.

Hardtmuth, T. (2011). *In der Dämmerung des Lebendigen – Hintergründe zu Demenz, Depression und Krebs* [In the Twilight of the Living – Background to Dementia, Depression and Cancer]. Heidenheim: Amthor Verlag.

Hardtmuth, T. (2017). *Medizin im Würgegriff des Profits* [Medicine in the Stranglehold of Profits]. Heidenheim: Amthor Verlag.

Hardtmuth, T. (2020a). Autonomie und Gesundheit [Autonomy and health]. In B. Rosslenbroich (ed.), *Perspektiven zur Biologie der Freiheit: Autonomieentwicklung in Natur, Kultur und Landschaft* [Perspectives on the Biology of Freedom: Autonomy Development in Nature, Culture and Landscape]. Stuttgart: Verlag Freies Geistesleben.

Hardtmuth, T. (2020b). The Corona Syndrome: why fear is more dangerous than the virus. *New View* magazine, 95 (Spring): 12–22.

Hardtmuth, T. (2021). *Mikrobiom und Mensch. Die Bedeutung der Mikroorganismen und Viren in Medizin, Evolution und Ökologie – Wege zu einer systemischen Perspektive* [The Microbiome and the Human Being. The Importance of Microorganisms and Viruses in Medicine, Evolution and Ecology – ways to a Systemic Perspective]. Berlin: Salumed-Verlag.

Hardtmuth, T. (2022). *What Covid-19 Must Teach Us: Meeting Viruses with Fear or Informed Common Sense?* Stroud, Glos.: Interactions.

Heisenberg, W. (1969). *Der Teil und das Ganze. Gespräche im Umkreis der Atomphysik* [The Part and the Whole. Conversations in the Field of Atomic Physics]. München: Piper Verlag.

Hontschik, B. & Maio, G. (2014). *Geschäftsmodell Gesundheit: Wie der Markt die Heilkunstabschafft.* [The Business of Health: How the Market Destroys the Art of Healing]. Berlin: SuhrkampVerlag.

House, R. & Loewenthal, D. (eds) (2008a). *Against and for CBT: Towards a Constructive Dialogue?* Ross-on-Wye: PCCS Books.

House, R. & Loewenthal, D. (eds) (2008b). CBT in Question: Special issue of *European Journal of Psychotherapy and Counselling,* 10 (3).

Hume, E.D. (2017). *Béchamp or Pasteur?: A Lost Chapter in the History of Biology.* A Distant Mirror (https://adistantmirror.com) (orig. publ. 1923).

Illich, I. (1976). *Limits to Medicine: Medical Nemesis – The Expropriation of Health.* Harmondsworth: Penguin,

Jonas, H. (2011). *Das PrinzipLeben* [The Principle of Life]. Berlin: SuhrkampVerlag.

Kaplan, H., Thompson, R.C., Trumble, B.C. & others (2017). Coronary atherosclerosis in indigenous South American Tsimane: a cross-sectional cohort study. *Lancet*, 389 (10080): 1730–9. Summary available at https://tinyurl.com/yc858y8u (accessed 5 May 2022).

Karlen, A. (1995). *Plague's Progress: A Social History of Man and Disease.* London: Orion.

Kashtan, M. (2017). Why patriarchy is not about men. Available at https://tinyurl.com/y2xldlc3 (accessed 2 October 2021).

Kentikelenes, A. & others (2014). Greece's health crisis: from austerity to denialism. *Health Policy*, 383 (9918): 748–53; *Lancet*, 22 February 2014.

Kidd, I.J. (2013). A pluralist challenge to 'integrative medicine': Feyerabend and Popper on the cognitive value of alternative medicine. *Studies in History and Philosophy of Biological and Biomedical Science*s, 44: 392–400.

Kidd. I.J. (2017). Reawakening to wonder: Wittgenstein, Feyerabend, and scientism. In J. Beale & I.J. Kidd (eds), *Wittgenstein and Scientism* (pp. 101–15). Abingdon, Oxon: Routledge.

Kidd, I.J. (2021). Feyerabend, science, and scientism. In K. Bschir & J. Shaw (eds), *Interpreting Feyerabend: Critical Essays* (pp. 172–90). Cambridge: Cambridge University Press.

Kidd, I.J., with House, R. & Brooks, O. (2021). The Long Interview: 'We're all Feyerabendians now!': Where Science and Society Meet – The Contemporary Relevance of Paul K. Feyerabend, 1924–94. *AHP Magazine for Self & Society*, 6 (Winter); available at https://tinyurl.com/bdh4hus4 (accessed 4 July 2022).

Kreiß, C. (2015). *Gekaufte Forschung – Wissenschaft im Dienst der Konzerne* [Purchased Research – Science at the Service of the Corporations]. Berlin: Europa Verlag.

Kuhn, T.S. (1962). *The Structure of Scientific Revolutions*. Chicago:

Chicago University Press (2nd edition, 1970).

Lange, M. (2016). Genom in Aufruhr: Der Mensch ist genetisch instabil [Genome in turmoil: Humans are genetically unstable]. Cologne: Deutschlandfunk Radio Station, 4 December; available at https://tinyurl.com/3ypy48b4 (accessed 2 June 2022).

Layard, R. (2011). *Happiness: Lessons from a New Science* (2nd edn). Harmondsworth: Penguin.

Layard, R. & Ward, G. (2020). *Can We Be Happier?: Evidence and Ethics.* Harmondsworth: Pelican.

Legewie, H. & Trojan, A. (nd). Theorie und Forschung zur Gesundheitsförderung [Theory and research for promotion of health]; available at https://tinyurl.com/mr36rmc6 (accessed 5 May 2022). Adapted from Trojan & Legewie (2000).

Lester, D. & Parker, D. (2019). *What Really Makes You Ill? Why Everything You Thought You Knew about Medicine is Wrong.* Independently published, ISBN 978-1673104035.

Light, D.W. (2014). The epidemic of sickness and death from prescription drugs. *ASA Footnotes*, 42 (8); available at https://tinyurl.com/6u633zwt (accessed 19 September 2021).

Light, D.W., Lexchin, J. & Darrow, J.J. (2013). Institutional corruption of pharmaceuticals and the myth of safe and effective drugs. *Journal of Law, Medicine and Ethics*, 14 (3): 590–610; available at https://tinyurl.com/pa67nfp6 (accessed 19 September 2021).

Lütge, C. & Esfeld, M. (2021). Und die Freiheit?: Wie die Corona-Politik und der Missbrauch der Wissenschaft unsere offene Gesellschaft bedrohen. [And Freedom?: How Corona Politics and the Abuse of Science Threaten Our Open Society]. Munich: Riva.

McGrath, L., Griffin, V., Mundy, E. & others (nd). The psychological impact of austerity: a briefing paper. UK: Psychologists Against Austerity; available at https://tinyurl.com/y36cttsz (accessed 9 August 2021).

McGrath, L., Griffin, V., Mundy, E. & others (2016). The psychological impact of austerity: a briefing paper. *Educational Psychology Research and Practice*, 2 (2): 46–57; available at https://tinyurl.com/5c6ajtkz (accessed 2 June 2022).

Madden, K.S., Szpunar, M.J. & Brown, E.B. (2013). Early impact of social isolation and breast tumor progression in mice. *Brain, Behavior, and Immunity*, 30 (Suppl), March: 135–41. Available at https://tinyurl.com/5n7833d7 (accessed 5 May 2022)

Maio, G. [date unknown]. Wider die okonomisierte Medizin [Against economised medicine]. *Forschung & Lehre*, 4/13: 261; available at https://tinyurl.com/4tzh8c34; accessed 5 May 2022.

Maio, G. (2014). *Geschäftsmodell Gesundheit – wie der Markt die Heilkunst abschafft* [Health – how the market is abolishing the art of healing]. Berlin: Suhrkamp Verlag.

Martin, L.H., Gutman, H. & Hutton, P.H. (eds) (1998). *Technologies of the Self: A Seminar with Michel Foucault*. Amherst, Mass.: University of Massachusetts Press.

Mencken, H.L. (1918/1923). *In Defense of Women*. Available at https://tinyurl.com/4tx4xu2jm (accessed 5 May 2022).

Meschnig, A. (2021). Die Corona-Impfung als Kommunion [The Corona vaccine as communion]. Achgut.com, 13 July; available at https://tinyurl.com/59fce654 (accessed 2 June 2022).

Metzinger, T. (2009). *The Ego Tunnel: The Science of the Mind and the Myth of the Self*. New York: Basic Books.

Moustafa, A., Xie, C., Kirkness, E. & others (2017). The blood DNA virome in 8,000 humans. *Public Library of Science (PLOS) Pathogens*, 13 (3): e1006292; available at https://tinyurl.com/2p9pmsz8 (accessed 2 June 2022).

Peters, E. (2020). Wie die Haut den Stress reguliert. [How the skin regulates stress]. In C. Schubert & M. Singer (eds), *Das Unsichtbare hinter dem Sichtbaren. Gesundheit und Krankheit neu denken* [The Invisible behind the Visible. Rethinking Health and Disease], pp. 79–107. Norderstedt: Books on Demand / Herstellung und Verlag.

Popper, K.R. (1963). *Conjectures and Refutations: The Growth of Scientific Knowledge*. London: Routledge & Kegan Paul.

Preston, J., Munevar, G. & Lamb, D. (eds) (2000). *The Worst Enemy of Science? Essays in Memory of Paul Feyerabend*. Oxford: Oxford University Press.

Rißmann, Dr W. & Pflug, C. (nd). Unsere Angst: Interview mit Dr. med. Wolfgang Rißmann, Psychiater. [Our fear: Interview with Dr. medical Wolfgang Rissmann, psychiatrist]. Available at https://tinyurl.com/28ne9dxe (accessed 5 May 2022).

Rosa, H. (2020). Unverfügbarkeit [Unavailability]. See https://tinyurl.com/2p9vats7 (accessed 5 May 2022).

Ross-Williams, R.L. (2020). Fear is stress that causes weakening of the immune system. *Journal of Clinical Cases and Reports*, 3 (S4): 19–21; available at https://tinyurl.com/3uxd8tsz (accessed 19 September 2021).

Rosslenbroich, B. (ed.) (2020). *Perspectives on the Biology of Freedom*. Stuttgart: VerlagFreiesGeistesleben.

Ryan, F. (2010). *Virolution – die Macht der Viren in der Evolution*

[Virolution – the Power of Viruses in Evolution]. Heidelberg: Spektrum Akademischer Verlag 2010.

Schad, W. (2014). *Der periphere Blick: Die Vervollständigung der Aufklärung* [The Peripheral View: Completing the Enlightenment]. Stuttgart: Freies Geistesleben.

Scheurle, H.J. (2016). *Das Gehirn ist nicht einsam: Resonanzen zwischen Gehirn, Leib und Umwelt* [The Brain Is Not Lonely: Resonances between the Brain, Body and Environment]. Stuttgart: W. Kohlhammer Verlag.

Schubert, C. & Amberger, M. (2016). *Was uns krank macht – was uns heilt: Aufbruch in eine neue Medizin. Das Zusammenspiel von Körper, Geist und Seele besser verstehen* [What makes us sick – what heals us: Departure into a new medicine. Better understand the interplay of body, mind and soul]. Munderfing: Fischer & Gann Verlag.

Sharpe, V.A. & Faden, A.I. (1998). *Medical Harm: Historical, Conceptual, and Ethical Dimensions of Iatrogenic Illness.* Cambridge: Cambridge University Press.

Shiva, V. (1993). *Monocultures of the Mind: Perspectives on Biodiversity and Biotechnology.* London: Zed Books.

Sinason, V. (1995). Review of Erskine & Judd, 1994. *Journal of Child Psychotherapy*, 31 (1): 131–3.

Sorgner, H. (2016). Challenging expertise: Paul Feyerabend vs. Harry Collins & Robert Evans on democracy, public participation and scientific authority. *Studies in History and Philosophy of Science*, Part A, 57 (June): 114–20.

Spitzer, M. (2018). *Einsamkeit. Die unerkannte Krankheit* (Loneliness – the Unrecognized Disease). Munich: Droemer & Knaur Verlag.

Standring, A. & Davies, J. (2020). From crisis to catastrophe: the death and viral legacies of austere neoliberalism in Europe?' *Dialogues in Human Geography*, 10 (2): 146–9; available at https://tinyurl.com/y4rj3nps (accessed 19 September 2021).

Stein, H.S. (1985). *The Psychodynamics of Medical Practice: Unconscious Factors in Patient Care.* Berkeley: University of California Press.

Steiner, R. (2009). *Das Hereinwirken geistiger Wesenheiten in den Menschen: Dreizehn Vorträge, gehalten in Berlin zwischen dem 6. Januar und 11. Juni 1908* [The Influence of Spiritual Beings in People: Thirteen Lectures held in Berlin, 6 January – 11 June 1908], GA 102. Dornach, Switzerland: Rudolf Steiner Verlag. Also available at https://tinyurl.com/2zhsrkmc (accessed 5 May 2022).

Steiner, R. & Wegman, I. (1991). *Grundlegendes für eine Erweiterung der Heilkunst* [Fundamentals for an Extension of the Art of Healing] (GA

27). Dornach, Switzerland: Rudolf Steiner Verlag.

Tarnas, R. (1991). *The Passion of the Western Mind: Understanding the Ideas that Have Shaped Our World.* New York: Ballantine.

Tavris, C. & Aronson, E. (2015). *Mistakes Were Made (But Not by Me): Why We Justify Foolish Beliefs, Bad Decisions, and Hurtful Acts,* 3rd edn. London: Pinter and Martin.

Taylor, G.J. (1989). *Psychosomatic Medicine and Contemporary Psychoanalysis.* Madison, CT: International Universities Press.

Technische Universität Berlin (2020). Willkommen beim ZTG: Technik und Gesellschaft im Zentrum - 20 Jahre gelebte Inter- und Transdisziplinaritat [Welcome to the ZTG: Technology and society at the centre – 20 years of lived inter- and transdisciplinary work]. Available at https://tinyurl.com/353uztsd (accessed 2 July 2022).

Trojan, A. & Legewie, H. (2000). *Nachhaltige Gesundheit und Entwicklung – Leitbilder, Politik und Praxis der Gestaltung gesundheitsförderlicher Umwelt- und Lebensbedingungen* [Sustainable Health and Development – Guiding Principles, Policies and Practices of the Design of Health-promoting Environmental and Living Conditions]. Frankfurt: Verlag für Akademische Schriften.

Vlachadis, N. & others (2014). Mortality and the economic crisis in Greece. *Lancet,* 383, 22 February: 691.

Vollmann, J. (2013). Persönlicher – besser – kostengünstiger? Kritische medizinethische Anfragen an die 'personalisierte Medizin' [More personal, better and cheaper? A critical analysis of 'personalised medicine']. *Ethik in der Medizin,* 25: 233–41; summary available at https://tinyurl.com/yc8428rd (accessed 5 May 2022).

Warden, M. (2021). 5G and coronaviris: an interim report. *New View* magazine, 101 (Oct–Dec): 45–9.

Wilkinson, R. & Pickett, K. (2016). *Equality. Warum gerechte Gesellschäften für alle besser sind.* Berlin: Verlag Haffmans & Tolkemitt. (English edn: *The Spirit Level: Why Greater Equality Makes Societies Stronger.*)

Wilmanski, T., Diener, C., Rappaport, N. & others (2021). Gut microbiome pattern reflects healthy ageing and predicts survival in humans. *Nature Metabolism,* 3 (2): 274–86.

Zeh, J. (2010). *Corpus Delicti: Ein Prozess.* [Corpus Delicti: A Trial]. Munich: Btb Verlag.

Zittlau, J. (2021). Good is what changes. *Die Welt,* 6 April.

Index

cattle farms: ecosystem of, 69
causal thinking/attributions, 55;
    mechanistic conceptions, 72;
    rethinking, 71
CBT: *see* Cognitive Behaviour Therapy
centrifugal thinking, 67
Černič, M., 63
chemotherapy treatment, 29, 58;
    senseless, 36
civil liberties, 18
Cognitive Behaviour Therapy, 118
cognitive dissonance, 89
Cohen, F., 79
collectivism, return of (Esfeld), 115
commercialisation of health care, 27–30
complementary medicine, 44, 106–7
Confronting the Experts (Martin), 40n
Conjectures and Refutations (Popper), 40
consciousness: evolution of, 73; -soul, age
    of, 14, 63
'conspiracy theory' narratives, 45
conversion, 109–10
Corona crisis, 11–13 *passim*, 26; collateral
    damage, 82; and inequality, 25; *see
    also* Corona measures, Covid-19
Corona measures: long-term
    consequences of, 99
'Corona vaccination as communion, The'
    (Meschnig), 85
coronary calcifications, 98
Corpus delicti (Zeh), 112
Covid-19, 17; 5G technology and, 95;
    damaging regulations, 79; dying from,
    85; hysteria, 91–7 *passim*; long-term
    immunological effects, 81; 'pandemic',
    80; *see also* Corona crisis
cow: as sacred animal, 70
critical journalism: failure of, 38–9
Crook, J., 73
crowd formation: *see* Mass Formation
cytoplasm, 76(n)

Das Prinzip Leben (Jonas), 76
Davies, J., 79
Davis, Professor Mark Morris, 16
death: causes of, 22; uni-causal
    explanations of, 85; *see also* death

anxiety, dying with
death anxiety: deployment of, 87; and
    terror, 92
debt crisis, 26
deforestation, 32; and Ebola epidemics,
    31
delusional narratives, 90
depression, 124
Der Mensch als Holobiont (Bosch), 74
deregulation of financial markets, 24, 25,
    27
Descartes, René, 15
Desmet, Mattias, 45n, 86, 90–4 *passim*,
    100
determinism, 55–6, 123–4
Deutsch, Felix, 72, 109
development: universal potential for, 121
diagnosis, 107–9, 111, 117
Dineen, T., 87
disease: stress-associated, 18; *see*
    autoimmune disease, illness, infectious
    diseases
disproportionality, 92
diversity: dynamic, 70; loss of, 26–7; *see
    also* microbial biodiversity
doctor–patient relationships, 117
Dodsworth, L., 80, 96
Domschke, Katharina, 59
drama triangle (Karpman's), 86, 87(n)
dualistic worldview, 15, 73; overcoming
    the, 77; *see also* Cartesian paradigm
Dürr, Hans Peter, 75, 121
dynamic concept of health, 101, 110
dynamic diversity, 70
dying with: vs dying from, 85; *see also*
    death

Ebola epidemics: deforestation and, 31
ecological crisis, 30–5
education: von Humboldt on, 57n
ego-forces, 51, 122
EHEC (*enterohaemorrhagic Escherichia
    coli*), 69n
electromagnetic radiation, 17; *see also* 5G
    technology
Empedocles, 74(n)
enemy image of micro-organisms/viruses,

Martin, Brian, 40n
Martin, Eric C., 43n
Martin, L.H., 118
mask-wearing, 93; child, 34
Mass Formation (Desmet), 45n, 91–7
    passim, 100
mass hypnosis, 91; *see also* Mass
    Formation
mass media: opinion management, 27;
    violence-glorifying, 38
mass vaccinations: *see* vaccinations
materialism: dogma of, 55; metaphysical
    assumptions of, 42
meaning: pervasive lack of, 91
media: 'good lies' in the, 96;
    manufacturing fear, 96; and Mass
    Formation, 92; psycho-techniques,
    35–40; *see also* mass media
medical research, 119: methodological
    constraints of, 58
medical training, 117, 122; university
    conformity, 122
medicalisation of society, 29
medications: lucrative long-term, 98
medicine: anthroposophical, 44, 53; battle
    mentality in, 62; commercialisation
    of, 28, 119, 124–5; complementary,
    44, 106–7; degradation of, 119;
    disastrous fusion with economics,
    60, 119; environmental, 72; etheric,
    53; functional, 72; holism in, 109;
    iatrogenic, 106; integral, 58, 100;
    personal relationship with a, 59;
    personalised, 120; person-centred, 72;
    postmodern, 71; preventive, 98–9;
    psychosomatic, 52n, 72, 109, 117;
    talking, 123
Meijer, D., 17n
Mencken, H.L., 87–8
mental states: gut bacteria and, 74
Meschnig, Alexander, 85
Metzinger, T., 121
microbial biodiversity: loss of, 33
microbiome, 19, 20, 21, 32–4, 76–7, 101,
    102, 121; gut, 33; individualisation of,
    113–14; loss of diversity, 20, 33–34;
    research, 63; unique intestinal, 59

micro-organisms: co-evolution with, 75;
    enemy image of, 19–22, 62
Mistakes Were Made (But Not by Me)
    (Tavris & Aronson), 89–90
Mölling, Karin, 74
money: as end in itself, 23
monocultures, 70: of the mind (Shiva),
    65; pathology of, 65
mosquitoes: Anopheles, 32
Moustafa, A., 64
'mysterious leap from mind to body'
    (Deutsch), 72, 109–10

National Health Service (UK), 28
NATO: eastward expansion of, 37
natural science: vs the humanities, 77
nature: deep mistrust of, 70; Heisenberg
    on, 77; unlimited biodiversity of, 105
neoliberal economics, 53–4, 57
neurodermatitis, 102
neurotransmitters, 12
NHS: *see* National Health Service
nucleotides, 104

Olivero, J., 31
Olson, S.H., 32n
ontology: defined, 66n
organic agriculture, 32
Oxfam study on inequality, 25(n)

pandemic: of fear, 61; as business model,
    54; and polarisation, 7
panpsychism, 72
Paracelusus, 74(n)
paradigm shift, 7–8
Parker, David, 43
parvoviruses, 64n
Pasteur, Louis, 62
'pathological imprinting', 34
patriarchy, 66
PCR test, 111
peripheral view (Schad), 67
personalised medicine: limitations of, 120
Perspektiven einer Biologie der Freiheit
    (Rosslenbroich), 50
Peters, E., 103
pharmaceuticals: lobby, 39n; toxic, 29

About the authors

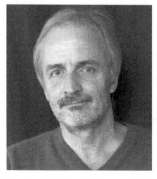

THOMAS HARDTMUTH, MD, studied human medicine at the TU and LMU Munich between 1978 and 1985. He trained as a consultant surgeon at Heidenheim Hospital and as a thoracic surgeon at Ulm University Hospital, and between 1996 and 2016 was senior physician at Heidenheim Hospital. From 2011 to 2020, Thomas was Lecturer in Health Sciences, Epidemiology and Social Medicine at the Baden-Württemberg Cooperative State University, and he also trained as a Waldorf school teacher while working. For many years he was involved in the working group 'Projects of Goethean Science' at the Carl Gustav Carus Institute in Öschelbronn and in the microbiology working group at the Goetheanum in Dornach/Switzerland. Other main research interests are neurobiology, oncology, health economics and the autonomy principle in salutogenesis.

For many years Thomas has regularly given lectures and seminars, and has published on various topics, mainly in the medical field.

Book publications:

Das verborgene Ich – Aspekte zum Verständnis der Krebskrankheit,
    Amthorverlag, Heidenheim, 2003
Denkfehler – das Dilemma der Hirnforschung, Amthorverlag,
    Heidenheim, 2006
*In der Dämmerung des Lebendigen – Hintergründe zu Demenz,
    Depression und Krebs*, Amthorverlag, Heidenheim, 2011
*Medizin im Würgegriff des Profits – die Gefährdung der Heilkunst
    durch die Gesetze der Ökonomie*, Amthorverlag, Heidenheim,
    2017
Mikrobiom und erweiterter Organismusbegriff, in *Jahrbuch für
    Goetheanismus*, 2017

The role of viruses in evolution and medicine – attempt at a systemic perspective, in *Jahrbuch für Goetheanismus*, 2019

Autonomy and health and 'Is a horse a work of art?' – On the aesthetic in evolution, in B. Rosslenbroich (ed.), *Ideas on the Biology of Freedom*, Stuttgart, 2020

The Corona syndrome: why fear is more dangerous than the virus, in C. Eisenstein, T. Hardtmuth, C. Hueck & A. Neider, *Corona and the Overcoming of Separateness*, Stuttgart, 2020

Microbiome and Humans: The Significance of Microorganisms and Viruses in Medicine, Evolution and Ecology – Paths to a Systemic Perspective, Salumed-Verlag, Berlin, 2021

What Covid-19 Must Teach Us: Meeting Viruses with Fear or Informed Common Sense, InterActions, Stroud, 2022

Das Virom des Menschen – Systembiologische Argumente gegen ein altes Feindbild sowie Medienpsychologische Aspekte zur Coronakrise, in M. Glöckler (ed.), A. Neider (ed.), *Corona – was uns die Pandemie lehren kann*, Stuttgart, 2022.

Several of Thomas' articles have also appeared in the cultural journal *die Drei* (see http://diedrei.org/autoren-anzeigen/autor/hardtmuth-thomas.html) as well as in *Elemente der Naturwissenschaft* (https://elementedernaturwissenschaft.org/en).

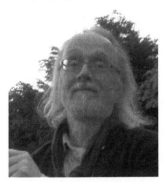

RICHARD HOUSE, MA [Oxon], Ph.D. is a chartered psychologist and freelance educational consultant/campaigner in Stroud, UK. He was previously a Senior Lecturer in Early Childhood at the University of Winchester (2012–14) and lectured in psychotherapy and psychology at the University of Roehampton from 2005 to 2012. Richard is editor of *Self and Society: International Journal for Humanistic, Existential and Transpersonal Psychology,* and he is a founding member of the Independent Practitioners Network and the Alliance for Counselling and Psychotherapy. He is a trained Steiner kindergarten and classroom teacher and has published several books on education – most notably, *Too Much, Too Soon? Early Learning and the Erosion of Childhood* (editor, Hawthorn Press, 2011), *Childhood, Well-being and a Therapeutic Ethos* (Karnac/Routledge, 2009; edited with Del Loewenthal), and

Pushing back to Ofsted (Interactions, 2020).

Richard was a founding member of the 'Open EYE' Campaign, Early Childhood Action and the Save Childhood Movement, and he organised the three press Open Letters on the state of modern childhood in 2006, 2007 (both with Sue Palmer) and 2011 in the *Daily Telegraph.* Between 1990 and 2007 Richard practised as a counsellor/psychotherapist and supervisor in general medical practice and privately, and he has published several hundred articles, academic papers, book reviews and book chapters in the literature on a wide range of subjects.

His current interests include the 'audit culture' in education and in society more generally; the psychodynamics of learning and teaching; post-structuralist and trans-modernist approaches to knowledge; critical perspectives on technology and technocracy; discourses on the 'new world order'; and the work of Rudolf Steiner and Paul Feyerabend. Richard has a particular current interest in the philosophy of science, and contesting medical and healing paradigms.

Books on psychotherapy and counselling:

Implausible Professions: Arguments for Pluralism and Autonomy in Psychotherapy and Counselling, PCCS Books, 1997; 2nd edn, 2011 (edited with N. Totton)

Therapy Beyond Modernity: Deconstructing and Transcending Profession-centred Therapy, Karnac Books, 2003

Ethically Challenged Professions: Enabling Diversity and Innovation in Psychotherapy and Counselling, PCCS Books (edited with Y. Bates)

Against and For CBT: Towards a Constructive Dialogue? PCCS Books, 2008 (edited with D. Loewenthal)

Compliance? Ambivalence? Rejection? – Nine Papers Challenging HPC Regulation, Wentworth Learning Resources, 2009 (edited with D. Postle)

Critically Engaging CBT, Open University Press, 2010 (edited with D. Loewenthal)

In, Against and Beyond Therapy: Critical Essays Towards a 'Post-professional' Era, PCCS Books, 2010

Humanistic Psychology: Current Trends and Future Prospects, Routledge, 2017 (edited with D. Kalisch and J. Maidman)

Acknowledgements

Thomas would like to thank Leandra Weckardt and Felix Hardtmuth for their contribution to the cover design, Erich Schneeweiß for his careful editing of the German edition, and Eva Amthor and Bernhard Masur from Amthorverlag for their friendly and good co-operation. My special thanks go to Richard House for the idea for this project and for his adept and sensitive way of conducting the dialogue, additionally for his careful editing of the English edition. On behalf of all courageous and committed truth-seekers, I would like to express my sincere appreciation for his valuable work.

Richard would like to thank in particular his co-author Thomas (Hardtmuth) for entering so whole-heartedly into this project with such eagerness, commitment and expertise; and Richard Brinton for his faith in the project and his willingness to publish its fruits. Richard models the patience and vision exemplified by all great publishers.

More generally, we will always be grateful to those great writers and researchers on health and well-being, going back many years, on whose shoulders we stand, and who have had the courage to speak medical and scientific truth to power, wherever it might lead.

Further titles by InterActions

https://interactions360.org

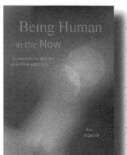

BEING HUMAN IN THE NOW:
Conversations with the soul of my sister Ajra

by Ana Pogacnik

2022. ISBN 978-9528364-6-9 UK £12
Pb 120 pp. With illustrations.

Ten years after her death, the author takes up conversations with the soul of her departed sister, revealing profound insights into challenges humanity is facing. The themes covered are direct, detailed and breathtakingly lively and highly topical, from the increasing difficulties souls have in crossing the threshold, to current topics affecting this, including suicides, medications and the dangers of the new mRNA vaccinations with their ability to penetrate the 'divine script' of our body. Inspiring are the descriptions of the deep significance of love as a source of strength, and of the spiritually radiating living being we know as earth which we can learn to interact with. In all of this the message is: the departed souls are eager to work more closely with us, bringing healing and fertilisation for the present and future.

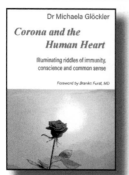

CORONA AND THE HUMAN HEART:
Illuminating riddles of immunity, conscience and common sense

by Michaela Glöckler, MD
Foreword by Branko Furst, MD

2021. ISBN 978-0-9528364-5-2, UK £7.95
Pb 96 pp, colour and B&W illustrations,

New inspiring research on the significant role of the heart in the development of the immune system and the importance this understanding has for health and for the Covid crisis. The author leads us on a path showing how, by strengthening our inner spiritual self — our inner sun — we will be strengthening our health and immunity, as well as illuminating riddles of conscience and common sense.

"This timely book represents a breakthrough in phenomenological research that will provide far-reaching insights..." B. Furst, M.D.

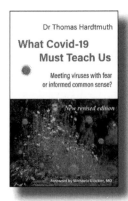

WHAT COVID-19 MUST TEACH US
Meeting viruses with fear or informed common sense?

by Thomas Hardtmuth, MD.
Foreword by Michaela Glöckler, MD.

2nd edition, 2022. ISBN 978-0-9528364-7-6
122 pages, £8.95

In this extended edition of the popular *What Covid-19 Can Teach Us*, Dr Hardtmuth provides a detailed and updated analysis of the multi-dimensional Corona crisis, with valuable insights relevant for any future health crisis. With evidence-based holistic perspectives, the author examines many intrinsically related topics including an in-depth description of our immune system resilience, the latest science recognising viruses not as 'enemies' but as vital for human evolution and health. They are a necessary part of a diverse intestinal microbiome. He examines further details around the Covid pandemic – what it *must* teach us for the future, including the use of PCR tests, risks of vaccinations during an epidemic, the significant impact of fear and negative publicity on immunity, and, importantly, the unhealthy relationship between politics, business and medicine.

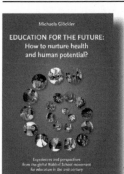

EDUCATION FOR THE FUTURE:
How to nurture health and human potential?

by Michaela Glöckler, MD.

2020. ISBN 978-0-9528364-3-8 UK £19.99
248 pages. Pb, colour photos and illustrations.

'Almost every day you can read somewhere that a fundamental change is needed in schools and the education system...' M.G.

Education for the Future is a plea for radically aligning upbringing and education with what is needed for the healthy development and well-being of children and adolescents. A unique contribution of Dr Glöckler is a year-by-year examination of human biological development and how this relates to soul-spiritual development, which in turn has a direct bearing on the needs of the child and what we can bring in the home and in education. It is the best prerequisite for a creative life into old age. A treasure chest of information and insights for educators, parents, carers and therapists alike.

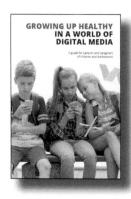

GROWING UP HEALTHY IN A WORLD OF DIGITAL MEDIA
A guide for parents and caregivers of children and adolescents

Written by specialists from 15 organisations concerned with media and childhood development. Introduction by Dr Michaela Glöckler.

2019. ISBN 9780 9528364 14, UK £10, 160 pages, sewn pb, colour illustrations and photos.

With increased screen use from Covid epidemic restrictions, this new guide is more relevant than ever. It explains child development considerations, noting dangers of inappropriate use and giving practical advice for a positive *age appropriate* use of digital media. It integrates a holistic approach, with consideration of physical, emotional and mental development of children. Easy to read. *An essential guide.*

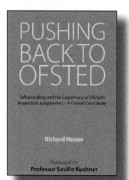

PUSHING BACK TO OFSTED
Safeguarding and the legitimacy of Ofsted's inspection judgements – a critical case study

by Richard House, Ph.D.
Foreword by Prof. Saville Kushner.
2020, ISBN 978-0-9528364-2-1, 128 pages. Pb. UK £10.99

'Ofsted' (Office for Standards in Education) in England is considered to be one of the harshest school inspectorates in the world. Dr House wrote this book following the closure of several Waldorf schools in the UK due to Ofsted inspections. He sets out in relentless detail the shortcomings and prejudices of the Ofsted report for one of those schools, as an example for how a state's one-size-fits-all approach can perpetuate a kind of violence on educational creativity and freedoms. It is a helpful study for any school facing intense state scrutiny and judgement. *"This analysis... is an uncomfortable but necessary challenge to current educational orthodoxies."* Dr Rowan Williams, former Archbishop of Canterbury.

Upcoming publication

(Provisional details – see website interactions360.org *for updates)*

LIMITS TO MEDICAL SCIENCE:
'Revolutionary' Conversations

edited by Richard House, Ph.D.

What happens when serious thinkers, academics and practitioners from a range of disciplines and professional backgrounds apply themselves to the machinations and complexities of modern health, illness and well-being, and co-create deep-dive conversations that interrogate the normally unarticulated assumptions underpinning the prevailing bio-medical paradigm? The result is *Limits to Medical Science* – a series of 'revolutionary' conversations which, taken together, lay the foundations for the new paradigm for human health that is so desperately needed, and the urgency of which the Covid era and its chronic medical mismanagement have thrown into sharp relief.

In this book of interview-dialogues conducted with Richard House, medical professionals, philosophers, psychologists and researchers ask the questions that mainstream medicine hardly ever addresses. Including major contributions from Professors Barrie Condon, Brian Martin, David Morris and Tom Sorell; Drs Martin Cohen, Thomas Hardtmuth, Ian James Kidd; and Psychologists and complementary health practitioners Vincent Di Stefano, Jill Hall and Dr Bruce Scott.

Anticipated publication in late 2022 /early 2023.

"**Beyond Mainstream Medicine** is a book I've long awaited. Allopathic medicine, sadly, has become fossilised around earlier beliefs rather than attuned to current research. What it once questioned it now takes as fact. The recent Covid crisis especially demonstrated this; according to a study by several US universities, Covid vaccines are more likely to put you in hospital than save you from it. Thomas Hardtmuth and Richard House not only illuminate philosophical and practice errors that undermine medicine, but suggest a way forward, which brings humanism and holistic vision inclusive of mind, body and spirit back into the medical fold. A must read for all public-facing health workers."

Professor Paul Barber (Ph.D.)
Bucharest, Romania

"Thomas Hardtmuth and Richard House agree that mainstream bio-pharmaceutical medicine is in need of urgent reform, if not a revolution. In this searching dialogue, they delve into the most fundamental assumptions and ontologies of illness, health and well-being, and offer pointers for how health systems need to change. Unmissable."

Dr Christian Buckland, Psychotherapist
Wokingham, UK

"This book by Thomas Hardtmuth and Richard House captures the spirit of the times. We urgently need a more humane medicine. A new medicine, in which the real human being with all his buried needs is seen in freedom and justice, in physical, soul and spiritual unity, in direct sensory perception, in social connectedness and in a higher consciousness, spiritually. I highly recommend **Beyond Mainstream Medicine**."

Univ.-Prof. Dr Dr Christian Schubert, Psychoneuroimmunologist
University of Innsbruck, Austria